Dr. Bob's Trans Fat Survival Guide

Why No-Fat, Low-Fat, Trans Fat is Killing You!

Robert DeMaria, D.C., N.H.D.
Director - Drugless Healthcare Solutions™

Laura A. Meyer, M.Ed.
ACSM Health and Fitness Instructor

Dr. Bob's Trans Fat Survival Guide

Why No-Fat, Low-Fat, Trans Fat is Killing You!

According to a study published in the Archives of Internal Medicine, men who eat a diet rich in trans fats have a higher risk of developing gallstones. In a recent 12-year follow-up study, 45,000 of these same male healthcare practitioners completed questionnaires about diet, medication, and health history with updates every 2 years. Their diets were evaluated every 4 years. The results of this study suggested that trans fats in the diet do indeed contribute to gallstones. What do you do with this information? Start by reading labels and subsequently eliminating all trans fats-known as hydrogenated and partially hydrogenated fats in ingredients listings from your diet. You'll be glad you did!

Robert DeMaria, D.C., N.H.D.
Director - Drugless Healthcare Solutions™

Laura A. Meyer, M.Ed.
ACSM Health and Fitness Instructor

Dr.Bob's Trans Fat Survival Guide

by Robert DeMaria, D.C., N.H.D.

Published by:

Drugless Doctor LLC™

362 East Bridge Street, Elyria, OH 44035
Phone: (440) 323-3841
Fax: (440) 322-2502
E-Mail: drbob@druglessdoctor.com
Web site: www.DruglessDoctor.com

Library of Congress Control Number: 2007906545
ISBN: 978-0-9728907-2-4

Printed in the United States of America
0 9 8 7 6 5 4 3 2

DISCLAIMER

This information is provided with the understanding that the author is not liable for the misconception or misuse of information included. Every effort has been made to make this material as complete and accurate as possible. The author of this material shall have neither liability nor responsibility to any person or entity with respect to any loss, damage or injury caused or alleged to be caused directly or indirectly by the information contained in this manuscript. The information presented herein is not intended to be a substitute for medical counseling.

Book Cover design by Peri Poloni-Gabriel, Knockout Design,
www.knockoutbooks.com

About Dr. Bob

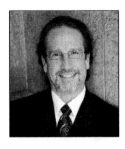

Dr. Bob has been extremely motivated over the last several years to orient his practice to helping those children who are becoming the pitiful products of the greed, ignorance, apathy and/or total lack of misunderstanding by the medical community, pharmaceutical companies, food manufacturers and parents who are too busy or in a total state of despair about what to do for their children. Dr. Bob has been trained and tested in utilization of nutritional and natural products. He has focused his attention on learning and seeking simple answers to tough questions. Patients of all ages– some with very bizarre histories and persistent conditions– continue to come to his office. These patients are treated with simple measures that, for whatever reason, medicine has ignored.

Beside a DC degree, Dr. Bob has a Bachelor's degree in human biology and is a consulting NHD. He has a Fellowship in Applied Spinal Biomechanical Engineering. He has taught in the legal, insurance, business and health care fields throughout the United States and in Europe. He has been an instructor at Oberlin College.

For over thirty years, Dr. Bob has treated thousands of patients using natural therapeutics. He has been trained to think independently where Western medicine so often limits health care providers into prescribing what the pharmaceutical companies are marketing at the time. He considers it a blessing to be an independent, self-employed health care provider who doesn't worry about pharmaceutical/ laboratory kick-backs and hospital jurisdiction. His ability to treat has not been hampered because of this and he continues to attract patients who need help.

When new patients present in his office, he never doubts that he can help that individual. He retraces habits from the beginning to find the root cause of problems–which a change of diet, spinal correction or the addition of basic supplements can correct. He treats patients the way God originally intended–naturally, without drugs.

This book is very exciting. It will change your life. Some of the information contained herein will be disturbing to some. But is works. Draw your line in the sand today. Have you had enough?

Peace and Blessings.
Dr. Bob

About Laura Meyer

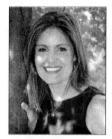 Laura Meyer earned a BA in English and spent 13 years in the classroom teaching English where she served as the Student Council Advisor and chairperson of the English department. Her commitment to health and fitness spurred her on to pursue her master's degree in Exercise Science where she utilizes her knowledge and skills as a personal trainer. Still not satisfied, she decided to also earn an American College of Sports Medicine Health and Fitness Instructor certification. She firmly believes everyone has the potential to achieve optimal health and feels that she can help others tap into that potential and, once and for all, attain their health and fitness goals. Laura is committed to natural health, believing that prevention is the first step to being healthy.

Laura also has an Ohio Nurses Association approved CEU curriculum, co-written with a colleague, which focuses on fitness for those in the high-stress nursing profession.

Besides teaching, writing, and training clients, Laura is mom to an awesome teenager who is an OSU Buckeye!

We want to thank you for obtaining a copy of our book!! With Dr. Bob's 30 plus years of experience in treating patients naturally and Laura's teaching experience in some form for nearly 15 years, that leads to 45 years of experience which we gladly pass on to you, our readers. The ideas presented in this book have been proven over years of trial and error. We know that once our ideas are implemented into your life, you will see healthy results. Read on; you'll be glad you did!!

Be Blessed.

Nutrition Facts

WARNING: Partially Hydrogenated Oils
(TRANS FAT) may be harmful to your family's health.

███████████████████████████████████

Amount Per Serving

Contents

███████████████████████████████████

INGREDENTS: Partially Hydrogenated oils (TRANS FAT),
any fat substitute. Always minimize these foods in your diet.

Preface

HOLD THAT FAT,
NEW YORK ASKS ITS RESTAURANTS
By MARC SANTORA
Article from the *New York Times*
Published: August 11, 2005

The New York City health department urged all city restaurants yesterday to stop serving food containing trans fats, **chemically modified ingredients that health officials say significantly increase the risk of heart disease and should not be part of any healthy diet.**

The request, the first of its kind by any large American city, is the latest salvo in the battle against fats, components of partially hydrogenated vegetable oils, three decades ago were promoted as a healthy alternative to saturated fats like butter.

Today, most scientists and nutrition experts agree that **trans fat is America's most dangerous fat** and recommend the use of alternatives like olive and sunflower oils.

"To help combat heart disease, the No. 1 KILLER in New York City, we are asking restaurants to voluntarily make an oil change and remove artificial trans fat from their kitchens," said Dr. Thomas R. Frieden, the city's health commissioner, who compared trans fats to asbestos and lead as public health threats. **"We are also urging food suppliers to provide products that are trans-fat free."**

It is far from clear how many restaurants will heed the call of Dr. Frieden, one of the city's most activist public health commissioners in a generation.

A survey by the department's food inspectors found that from 30 to 60 percent of the city's 20,000 restaurants use partially hydrogenated oil in food preparation, meaning that thousands of cooks and chefs might need to change their cooking and purchasing habits to meet the request. Trans fats are particularly prominent in baked goods, frying oils, and breading, and can be hard to replace without raising costs or changing the taste of familiar foods like cookies and French fries.

While the health department will not seek to ban the ingredient outright, it has begun an educational campaign among restaurateurs, their suppliers and the public denouncing trans fats. In a letter sent to all food suppliers in the city last week, Dr. Frieden wrote: "Consumers want healthier choices when eating out. Our campaign will increase consumer demand for meals without trans fat."

Many of the city's higher-priced restaurants already avoid using the fats, and Dr. Frieden said he had received a positive response from other restaurants and suppliers who will try to get on board.

"Working together to reduce trans fat from our kitchens will be one more way to ensure an enjoyable and healthy experience," said E. Charles Hunt, the executive vice president for the New York State Restaurant Association, which represents 7,000 restaurants across the state.

Public health officials contend that trans fat not only has the same heart-clogging properties as saturated fat, but also reduces the "good" cholesterol that works to clear arteries.

Denmark imposed a ban in 2003 on all processed foods containing more than 2 percent of trans fat for every 100 grams of fat. Canada is considering a similar ban.

Government agencies in the United States have been less interventionist, largely relying on the industry to police itself. Outside of New York, the only effort of note was a campaign in Tiburon, a small town in Marin County, Calif., that led to 18 local restaurants ending the use of trans fats.

New York's campaign comes on the heels of the Food and Drug Administration's finding that there is no safe level of trans fats in a healthy diet. As a result of that finding, all food companies must include trans fat levels in labeling information starting Jan. 1.

While the F.D.A. decision is already having a broad impact on processed foods sold in grocery stores, the city's effort will expand the campaign to include restaurants.

"Trans fat clearly contributes to heart disease, but it is something that is relatively new to the consumer environment," said Dr. Sonia Angell, the department's director of cardiovascular disease prevention and control.

Next year, the city plans to conduct another survey to determine the effectiveness of the campaign and will then assess what further steps might be needed.

While not naming individual restaurants, Dr. Angell said the survey the city recently completed did not show any clear patterns in terms of the types of places that use partially hydrogenated oil.

Among the alternatives available to replace partially hydrogenated oil, Dr. Angell said, are many common monounsaturated and polyunsaturated oils like olive, peanut, sunflower and cottonseed oils.

McDonald's and a few other fast food companies have pledged to use healthier alternatives to partially hydrogenated oils but have faltered in finding a solution that is both cost effective and that does not significantly alter the taste of their foods.

The city was careful to solicit the endorsement of the Restaurant Association before announcing its campaign, as well as the American Heart Association. However, many restaurant owners, workers and patrons interviewed yesterday greeted the city's campaign with some skepticism.

The reaction of Karen Quam, a waitress at the Bridgeview Diner in Bay Ridge, Brooklyn, was typical. "Labeling is as far as you want to go," she said. "You don't want to be telling people what to eat."

Dr. Frieden, stressing that the campaign was strictly voluntary, said he was optimistic that both the public and the industry would react positively to his appeal.

"I am aware of the changing winds regarding nutritional advice and therefore we have been very selective," he said.

He compared it to the situation with asbestos and lead, materials that at one point the public believed were safe but now are known to be dangerous. "In this case," he said, regarding trans fat, "the evidence is clear."

1

Introduction

Greetings!! I want to be the first one to congratulate you for obtaining this book of timely information. I have been saving, compiling, researching, analyzing, and reading about FAT since 1974 when I began my college studies. It is obvious that we live in an age where information for personal use is literally one click away. The content I see from my side of the mountain is not always told to us truthfully, accurately, or with clinically established results. Consumers who rely only on articles and news releases from questionable sources are being duped into believing everything in print. The pharmaceutical companies and health providers don't always release accurate information. Food manufacturers, drug producing companies, and the conventional health care machine in America have an enormous influence on what is **leaked** to the media. The public can be confused by the news releases we read: Eggs are Bad! Eggs are Good! Eat Low Fat to Lose Weight! Low Fat Makes You Fat! Aspirin is Good! Aspirin Causes Ulcers! WOW!! It is hard to decipher what to believe and what not to believe.

Micro pieces of information have been issued by the industry which financially benefits the most. I read the respected news sources extracting business trends and consumer appetites. With the conflicting information presented, it is obvious manufacturers today do not know exactly what the public wants. There is a measurable gap between those who live to eat and others who eat to live, the latter are aware that choices impact quantity and quality of life.

Look at America. It is estimated that over 60 percent of the population is obese. Obesity is now recognized as a disease. New vocabulary words have been added for this epidemic, terms like morbid obesity, gastric bypass, and liposuction. Who is to blame for this? I'm not sure and I don't believe we can point one finger at any one cause. But one thing of which I am sure: fat consumption is NOT the only reason for our waist and girth expansion.

Complicating the puzzle more are fabricated fats like trans or hydrogenated fats, made by heating vegetable oil and designed to be a replacement for lard, as well as other mutated man-made oils. What we need to understand is that heating oils to high temperatures twists and **distorts the chemical structure wreaking havoc in the cell membranes**. Not only are these oils altered due to heating them to high levels, but they are also used over and over again, some for long periods of time causing them to eventually become rancid. Over months and years ingesting these hydrogenated or trans fats, with their altered structural composition, does more harm to the body than consuming saturated animal and plant fats labeled as "bad." I am not denying that there is an ongoing debate on this saturated fat issue. I am not here to argue with any special interest group. I want to enhance your ability to make an educated decision on which fats you would like to include in your long-term health goals and which ones you will minimize because of their negative effects in your body.

I had restricted range of motion and pain in my neck and shoulder when I first came to see Dr. DeMaria. I began consuming organic foods and reduced or eliminated dairy, hydrogenated fats and sugar. Following Dr. Bob's advice and care has reduced my pain and increased my strength, energy and range of motion. Because of the honest information available through education, the patient is inspired and encouraged to take the primary active role in his healing and health maintenance rather than being an ill, ignorant, drug-dependent lemming.

~Kevin Gallagher

The perception and current thinking of the public is that there are good and bad fats. Red meat is categorized as a saturated fat which should be limited. Leaner sources of fat from meat like chicken and turkey are being encouraged instead. I know from experience that gravy made from the thick, slimy roast beef drippings found on the bottom of a baking dish with the addition of sugar-filled dessert will lead to a congested liver and a clogged vascular system.

Here is a thought to ponder: the public's education about red meat being bad and the likely cause of heart disease was introduced in the late 1940s. Until then, we ate beef regularly. My dad was raised by a single mom during the depression. His father died when he was nine. I believe his financial lack as a child and the global American prosperity post WWII created a pandemic societal feeding frenzy. Not only was there a chicken in every pot, but there was also roast beef being served every Sunday. In my home, beef-based meals led the way during the week — meatloaf, meat sauce, stroganoff, and whatever meal plan was found in the litany of ethnic household recipe boxes. Did beef consumption cause the problem, or did sugar loaded desserts at every meal and snack ever enter anyone's mind as a possibility for heart disease? Cardiovascular disease, CVD, which we will discuss in the next chapter, was the initial critical factor for all the fat hype we have to deal with today. I believe that the substitution of fats in the late 1970s from lard to hydrogenated fats and a multi-billion dollar surgical and cardiovascular industry, with all the peripherals — pharmaceutical companies, insurance companies — getting a piece of the action, is only a band aid to a problem that is beyond logical comprehension. Statistically, if 11 percent of the population changed their exercise and eating habits, the pharmaceutical and conventional health industries would have to change what they market. If these

> Statistically, if 11 percent of the population changed their exercise and eating habits, the pharmaceutical and conventional health industries would have to change what they market.

companies would reduce the production of aspirin, statin drugs, and defibrillators which drain the pockets of people with high health insurance costs and would market products that promote the quality of life, not just the longevity, they would go broke because society wouldn't need them any longer.

Do you realize that if your cholesterol is too low, your sexual function could be impaired?

I know that people are confused. Some of the health terminology we use today is neither true nor accurate. Cholesterol is not bad. It elevates as a protective response in the body. Do you realize that if your cholesterol is too low, your sexual function could be impaired? Did you know that while on cholesterol lowering medication, many have experienced decreased sexual desire? Advertisements on TV suggest that men today are having difficulty achieving erections. Pre-menopausal women are suffering from elevated estrogen symptoms (heavy menstrual flow, tender breasts, and uterine fibroids) which are directly related to progesterone deficiency. This in turn is created by the fast paced, daily grind which causes adrenal gland fatigue and cortisone deficiency resulting in a need for more cholesterol (see page 21) to make more cortisone to eliminate the pain because fibromyalgia has set in. That was a

---

Breast Cancer

In a study of more than 38,000 over-weight women, those with low HDL ('good') cholesterol (under 46 mg/dl) had roughly twice the risk of breast cancer of those with high HDL (over 63 mg/dl).

Researchers believe that low HDL is often a sign of insulin resistance, also called the metabolic syndrome. (Other signs are elevated levels of blood pressure, blood sugar, triglycerides, insulin, androgens or some other hormone that may raise the risk of cancer.)

What to do: If you're overweight, lose those extra pounds. (Low HDL wasn't linked to an increased risk of breast cancer in normal-weight women.) Exercise can help you slim down and — if you do enough — may raise your HDL.

J. Nat. Cancer Inst. 96: 1152, 2004

---

mouthful. All of this has been a result of being told that cholesterol is bad and we need statin drugs.

The human body is a self-healing unit. | I am a drugless healthcare provider and clinician. I assess and treat patients with chronic conditions and they improve without drugs. The human body is a self-healing unit. From my clinical based experience, medications should be used for a short season while the body is fed the right nutrients, cleansed of any toxins, and aligned posturally creating a state of correct alignment so vital information can be transmitted via the spinal cord to tissue cells and back. Medication has side effects, all of which are not life enhancing.

Regardless of your training, experience, or healthcare affiliation, physiology is physiology. The established medical community did not realize that fresh citrus (vitamin C) would prevent scurvy. Cleaning hands and utensils to prevent post-surgical infections was not immediately accepted. The powers that be at the time of Albert Einstein did not accept his theory of relativity because up to that point, discoveries were philosophically argued and proven versus being mathematically established. They could not dispute Einstein's theory logically.

Thomas Edison was another genius who created solutions to problems. Stories have been passed on that Edison on his discovery of the material used for the incandescent light bulb was questioned on the number of failed experiments he did to determine the perfect substance. He quickly responded that each experiment successfully eliminated an item not compatible for his hypothesis and eventually there was light!

You are living in a position of time and established scientific mindsets equal to the environment with which these past and awesome scientists had to contend. Our situation may be even more desperate because the ramifications of what will be discussed in this book and their ripple effect will have earth-shaking consequences. The general public in America is

I was bed-ridden or in a wheelchair for 1½ years due to a sporadic control of various muscles throughout my body. I was very foggy and unable to think clearly most of the time. Prior to being in a wheelchair, I took ibuprofen and allergy medications regularly. Also, antibiotics and anti-inflammatory drugs were taken frequently. I had also been on steroids, anti-depressants and something for auto-immune disease. The care and information from Dr. DeMaria saved my life! I believe I was on the path for far worse than a wheelchair had I not gone to his office. I had to modify everything. I received subluxation corrective care, whole food supplements, completely changed my diet, along with regular massages and colonics. I limited my schedule and commitments and even the way I handled and dealt with stress. I can't say that these changes weren't difficult because they were necessary. The alternative choice was to be in a wheelchair again and to not be able to think clearly. This motivator is what kept me going forward. The hardest change now is my time commitments. As I feel better, I want to do more and I have to be careful not to fall into that trap again.

I just want to say that prior to being in a wheelchair, I thought I was a normal individual with a hectic lifestyle and not so healthy eating habits, but nothing extremely bad. I had no idea that what I was doing to my body on the inside over all those years until my body gave up on me. Don't wait until your body gives up. Change your lifestyle before that happens!

~Cindy Bublenic

living quite desperate lives of poor health. Fear of cancer, Alzheimer's, stroke, diabetes, pain, and emotional distress are at pandemic levels. It was recently reported that nearly 50 percent of Americans take one prescription or more per month and 20 percent take three or more prescriptions per month. Close to 20 percent of Americans, about 50 million people, take anti-depressants which include warning labels saying the medication may cause death by suicide. That is not encouraging news. It has been estimated that anywhere from 130,000 to 160,000 people die every year from prescription drug mistakes equaling that of a full 747 jetliner crashing about

It has been estimated that anywhere from 130,000 to 160,000 people die every year from prescription drug mistakes equaling that of a full 747 jetliner crashing about every two days.

every two days. This estimate also equals the death toll from the 2004 tsunami disaster in Southeast Asia.

We have already been advised by the scientific community that up to 33 percent of currently healthy one- to three-year-olds will have diabetes in forty years due to poor health habits. Now there's a piece of information to lift your spirits. Do you think that the hierarchy in London during the 1650s told the merchant seamen at a union meeting that 50 percent of them would die if they went on the voyage without eating enough citrus fruits to prevent scurvy? My guess is, probably not.

Nuts to Diabetes

Women who ate nuts at least five times a week had a 30 percent lower risk of diabetes than women who almost never ate nuts in a study of more than 83,000 nurses. (Eating nuts one to four times a week or eating peanut butter at least five times a week was linked to a 20 percent lower risk.)

It's not clear whether nuts lower the risk of diabetes because they're high in magnesium, unsaturated fats, or fiber or whether something else about nut-eaters lowers their risk. The researchers took into account the fact that the nut-eaters ate healthier diets, were less likely to smoke and be over weight, and were more likely to exercise. But they may have missed something else about nut-eaters that made them healthier.

What to do: It's worth adding small servings of nuts to your diet; just keep in mind that they're calorie-dense, so you can't eat them without removing something else. (The study's authors recommend cutting out some refined grains and red meat.) You'll get 150 to 185 calories in a one-ounce serving of dry roasted nuts. That's just 22 almonds, or 14 walnut halves.

J. Amer. Med. Assoc. 288: 2554, 2002

The good news is that with modifying your diet to eliminate man-made fats, eating less food prepared in heated fat or oil regardless of the source, and taking whole food vitamins and minerals can help you stop, prevent, and in some situations, reverse your degeneration. Sound too good to be true? It is not!! Remember I am a drugless healthcare provider. I have not been trained to think in an "outside in" cause of disease. My training and mind set is to look for the cause physiologically, feed the body, detoxify the body, turn on the power supply through proper spinal alignment, and let the body heal itself from the inside out. Granted, some come too late, and their body is beyond repair, but the human will to live is far greater than we realize.

What will we be talking about over the next few pages? I want to easily describe to you what fat is and what it is not, how you deal with it, and how you make the necessary changes in your life to eliminate the bad fat. The terms and word pictures will be logical. I will not bore you with details of every equation, but there will be a Chemistry 101 section. I will offer some explanations of all the media hype surrounding "cox inhibitors." I also feel obligated to reveal the short comings of aspirin and why the patients — and I have seen thousands — I treat have no pain and have healthy heart function without aspirin. The role of essential fats in body health is not understood by health care providers in general. The masses are totally in the dark on what fats they should or should not consume. There is a pathway in the body where food becomes certain compounds necessary for life. These pathways, once understood, will give you a basis for your decisions, empowering your health future. The information provided to you will be honest and forthright. My motivation is in knowing that I have saved someone from unnecessary surgery or long term chemical dependency.

The information that I have received from Dr. DeMaria has changed my life. I had been dealing with numbness in my legs and arms with unsteadiness and fatigue. I also have MS and take prescription Avonex for the MS. By changing my diet (no sugar, no dairy, eating healthier and reducing stress) and taking the supplements suggested by Dr. Bob along with subluxation correction, I feel 1000 percent better. I now have more energy. I don't feel poorly any longer and this has led to a more positive mental outlook. Even with the MS, Dr. Bob has shown me how to work with my disorder and what is best for my situation in order to lead to a healthy, happy life.

~**Dave Page**

I am a son, dad and husband. As a son, I have seen my elderly parents become emotionally manipulated with fear tactics by their conventional healthcare providers. Being a dad has encouraged me, raising two outstanding young men in their twenties who lived their adolescent and teen lives without asthma, ADHD, eyeglasses, and cavities while excluding the help of medicine. Optimal female health teeters on a fine line of hormonal balance. My wife of thirty years made a quality decision about lifestyle modification when she was thirty and was diagnosed with cervical dysplasia and adult onset acne. She reset her food, beverage, and exercise choices and has been blessed with no female organ dysfunction or perimenopausal body signals. She has all her organs intact. As a baby-boomer male, I see and relate to the men in our society who have statistically stayed away from doctors. These men are in the same position I am in, plus many are divorced or single, raising children with or without cooperation or live with separation anxiety.

The very true reality when push comes to shove is, a majority of men **do not trust** the pill-pushing, out of touch, pharmaceutical healthcare system. I consistently see the "light go on" in my male patients' expressions when I explain to them how the body works and is self-healing when they follow the directions. They are aware that the many healthcare and pharmaceutical conglomerates are money motivated. The excitement radiates from them after they changed their lifestyle. They feel better faster than when they treated symptoms with medication. The enthusiasm of self directed health goal achievement surely must parallel the sailors' excitements on Christopher Columbus' ships when they beat the odds of the established, fear-thinking society and did not fall off the edge of the earth. We have been media-blasted that medicine is the only answer. Wake up!! There is a whole generation seeking alternative care and paying for it themselves. More people visit natural practitioners today than the conventional counterparts.

My dream is to shake up the status quo, raise the bar of health, and create a proactive public who demands affordable, quality, chemical- and toxic-free, non-GMO foods, water and air. Slowly the food manufacturers and even the fast food conglomerates are responding. Can you believe that McDonalds is one of the leading sellers of salads at 300 million annually? (Horovitz 2005) Whole Foods Market, a respected health food store network has 27 varieties of mixed greens. Kraft Foods is concerned that Frito-Lay, a pioneer company for removing transfat, is moving into the healthy snack food arena. (Terhune 2005) The consumers are making a ripple effect with their pocketbooks and wallets. (Ellison 2005) Wall Street is watching with concern. I am totally aware that the information presented will be unacceptable to those who have the most to lose financially. The information presented is time tested. It works. I have thousands of satisfied patients who are LIVING proof!! Be blessed. It's not over yet. You will get better naturally. Be patient and a student of natural therapeutics.

When I first came to see Dr. DeMaria I had very bad sinus problems. I was also taking blood pressure medication. The information provided by Dr. Bob has made me more aware of the value of what goes past my mouth and how it affects my entire body. I have greatly reduced my sugar intake and I also use flax oil daily along with fresh carrot juice. Yum! Staying away from processed food has been difficult. It is so easy to grab and eat, however I do not get any nutritional value from it. As a result from making a few lifestyle changes I hardly notice any problems at all! There are so many people who are my age at work with so many aches and pains due to their diet and I almost have none! I feel really good about my maintenance care from Dr. Bob.

~Rebecca Szilagyi

End Notes

Ellison, Sarah. "As Shoppers Grow More Finicky, Big Food Has Big Problems". *The Wall Street Journal.*

Horovitz, Bruce. "Salads Grow into Profitable Garden of Eatin." *USA Today.* January 24, 2005.

Terhune, Chad. "Frito-Lay to Refocus Marketing." *The Wall Street Journal.* February 25, 2005.

2

The Demise
of Fat

Cardiovascular disease, the bane of modern medicine, is the number one killer in the Western world. However, this was not always the case. In the early part of the 1900s, heart disease, today called cardiovascular disease, or CVD, was very rare resulting in only about six percent of all deaths in the United States. In 1947, Ancel Keys, Ph.D., a physiologist at the University of Minnesota, conducted a study of Minnesota professional men after noticing a peak in heart-related deaths in America. Prior to this study, Keys had spent the WWII years studying "starvation and subsistence diets" whose results were published in *Biology of Human Starvation*, 1950 (CDC, 1999). Keys noticed a sharp contrast between the deaths due to heart disease in the post-war European countries and the deaths due to heart disease in post-war America where starvation was not a way of life during WWII like it was in Europe. America was probably one of the best fed nations in the world. So, how deaths from heart disease could be occurring mystified Keys.

Since the American diet consisted of richer foods higher in animal fat in comparison to her European counterparts, it was easy for Keys to theorize that saturated fat was the culprit. So with the results from his Minnesota businessmen study and starvation studies in hand, Ancel Keys boldly claimed that "the diet of a population would be reflected in the level of cholesterol in the blood which, in turn, would affect susceptibility to coronary heart disease (CHD)" (Keys, 1980). Basically, that's all it took for our nation to jump on the no fat/low fat and no red meat or dairy bandwagons.

As the consumption of animal fat and cholesterol began to rise during this century, so did the incidence of CHD.

As the consumption of animal fat and cholesterol began to rise during this century, so did the incidence of CHD. People in most of the world have never increased their consumption of animal products. In these countries, CHD is still a rare illness (Ornish, 1982).

While Ancel Keys' postulation seemed both accurate and laudable to the average person, several important factors pertaining to CHD were ignored. First, during the 1930s, it was understood by "leaders in clinical medicine" that heart disease "is often caused by repeated infections, such as the common cold, which do injury to the organ." (Albert, 1927) It was an accepted thought that 15 percent to 25 percent of all cases of heart disease were due to rheumatic fever which people contracted during their childhoods. (Albert, 1927) Another point most ignored was that the Minnesota businessmen that Keys studied were wealthy. They ate richer foods than the average American could afford and were relatively inactive. Had Keys performed a study on middle-class Americans, the results would have been very different. Those people working long hours in manufacturing industries were also those who could not afford to eat a diet consisting of rich foods. What is interesting is that there are population groups who consume large amounts of fats and fatty foods while remaining incredibly free of heart diseases. The keys are in the types of fats consumed as well as other lifestyle factors.

Good for the Heart

People who eat beans, almond butter, and other legumes at least four times a week have a 21 percent lower risk of heart disease than those who eat legumes less than once a week, says a 19-year study of nearly 10,000 people.

The researchers couldn't say why bean-eaters have healthier hearts. Among the possibilities: beans have soluble fiber, which lowers cholesterol, and folate, which can lower blood levels of homocysteine, an amino acid that promotes heart disease.

What to do: Eat more beans. Think of them not as beans, but as chick pea curry, split pea soup, rice and lentils, burritos, hummus, and pasta e fagioli.

Arch. Intern. Med. 161: 2573, 2001

> **We have become a nation that is dependent on cholesterol and heart medications when our diets are the real culprits.**

We have become a nation that is dependent on cholesterol and heart medications when our diets are the real culprits. As you read the rest of this book, the goal is that you will see the importance of proper diet in our lives as a way to live healthier and more productive lifestyles and avoid long-term drug usage which eventually has a detrimental effect on our bodies.

End Notes

Albert, Dr. Henry. *Time Magazine*. October 23, 1927.

Ancel Keys, Ph.D. August 6, 1999. {online}. Available: http://www.cdc.gov/mmwr. (January 12, 2005)

Keys, Ancel. *Seven Countries: A Multivariate Analysis of Death and Coronary Heart Disease*. Harvard University Press, 1980.

Ornish, Dean. *Stress, Diet, and Your Heart*. New York: Holt, Rinehart and Winston, 1982.

3

Fat — Why and Why Not?

$\mathbf{F}$ood is essential for life. Man cannot survive without food. Americans love food. Look around. Families get together for dinners. Business meetings consist of snacks. We are not lacking sources of food. We have mega stores with endless rows of tasty morsels. Those endless rows are part of the dilemma; there's just too much food and not enough committed time to burn the excess. And I can't go without mentioning wrong fat consumption — man-made fat modification — industrial fat alteration — media fat misinformation — has created an enormous negative impact on our current level of healthy lifestyle existence.

People are dying, disabled, chemically dependent, surgically altered, and living in pain because of misunderstanding fat.

I am not totally convinced there is an easy answer for the magnitude of the problem we are facing. People are dying, disabled, chemically dependent, surgically altered, and living in pain because of misunderstanding fat. The socio-economic existence of our current medical system of patient care is largely fueled because of misinterpretation of cholesterol and fat. The pharmaceutical and conventional medical establishment generates billions, not millions, on lowering cholesterol levels to prevent heart attacks. Meanwhile, research suggests that it is inflammation of the vessels which creates heart attacks versus the elevated cholesterol level. Who do you believe? When did this all start? Why did this happen? What is the problem with trans fat anyway?

Here we go. Fat can be a challenging, hotly debated subject. I plan on keeping this logical and simple. Fat molecules are chains of carbon, like coal. Shared connections hold them together and are called bonds. Picture a row of children and every so often two are holding hands. That's a basic concept of a fat chain. The number of coal lumps in a row and how many pairs of held hands keeping the row in order determines the name and activity of the fat. The names of fats and their activities should be understood so you can make logical decisions on what to eat. Fats, like them or not, are incorporated into your body for fuel and to build cells, tissues, organs, hormones, etc.

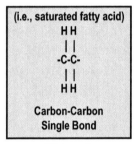

Figure 1

Saturated fat molecules are rows of carbons held together with one hand or bond (Figure 1). Saturated fats are solid at room temperature. They can also be from plant or animal sources although most are from animal sources. It has been suggested by many scientists that fat from animal sources is the major cause of our heart disease. Saturated fat, whether from plant or animal sources, was branded "bad" fat. These scientists correlated saturated fat with high cholesterol and heart disease. What is not commonly known is that saturated animal fat ALSO contains "healthy" monounsaturated fats and is in itself not bad, but is a part of a bigger problem.

About twenty years ago tropical oils with their saturated fat content were eliminated from most packaged food in favor of hydrogenated and partially hydrogenated fat. Now, advocates of plant-sourced, saturated fat, including palm and coconut oils, are suggesting that the properties and effects of their cholesterol free fat is not detrimental to health as once thought. Palm and coconut oils, from my observation, may in fact be a medium with which to cook food if you insist on frying your food. This is because heating saturated fat does not create partially-hydrogenated trans fat like heating vegetable oils does. Trans fat does occur in nature, but it does not impair health in this natural state. It is directly used as an energy source. The man-made, partially hydrogenated fat has a molecular carbon chain structure not compatible with natural cell interfacing.

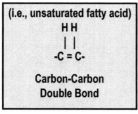

Figure 2

Monounsaturated fat molecules are chains of single bonded carbon with hydrogen and oxygen combinations linked together with at least one double bond or one pair of hands (Figure 2). This extra pair of hands creates a totally different set of possibilities. Monounsaturated fats are liquid at room temperatures and thicken in the refrigerator. The extra bond changes the flexibility of this molecule creating a more pliable and elastic versus a hard and stiff characteristic. An example of a monounsaturated fat is olive oil. It can be heated to moderate temperatures and is what I use to sauté food. Olive oil tastes great on a huge variety of foods on which you may normally put butter. Monounsaturated fats can have various lengths or coal lumps in their chains. There is a classification of monounsaturated fats called oleic acid. Oleic acid has its double bond position at the number nine or ten bond positions. It is found in olive, almond, pistachio, pecan, avocado, hazelnut, cashew and macadamia oils, as well as in the membranes of plant and animal cell structures. Oleic acid keeps arteries supple or soft. It resists damage by oxygen and therefore is stable. It melts at 55 degrees Fahrenheit. I wanted to bring this up because you may see this classification on future food labels.

An example of a monounsaturated fat is olive oil.

Oleic acid keeps arteries supple or soft.

Polyunsaturated fat molecules are made of chains of carbon atoms with single hydrogen and oxygen and is also connected by multiple, double=hand holding (Figure 3). Hence the name poly- or multiple unsaturation. These molecules are liquid. They do not get hard at room

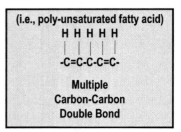

Figure 3

temperature and they remain liquid in cool environments. The multiple pairs of held hands, or double bonds, create a configuration where the molecules can actually bend upon themselves in a C, commonly called Cis position (Figure 4).

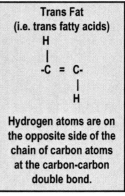

Figure 4

Figure 5

The man made, partially hydrogenated fat has a molecular carbon chain structure not compatible with natural cell interfacing. It is "T" shaped and disrupts cell membrane function (Figure 5). This is very important for you to know and will be discussed further in Chapter 8.

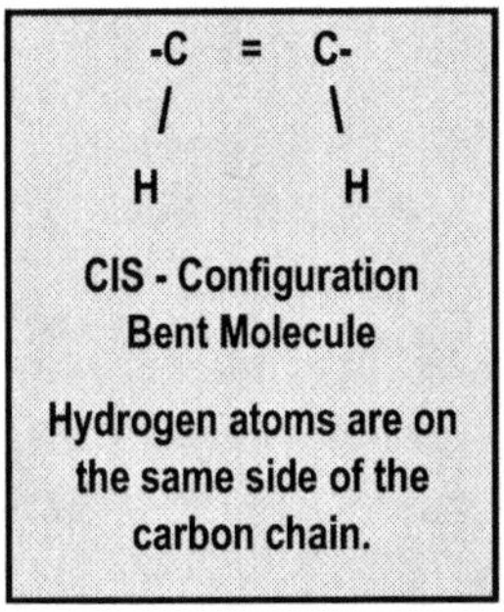

Imbalanced fat consumption with either a heavy focus on saturated and heated vegetable oils is what creates unhealthy bodies.

I have evidence based observations I want to clarify in order for you to get the Big Idea. Fats and oils found in nature, in the raw, uncooked state, are neither bad nor good. Heat adversely modifies fat molecules in mono and polyunsaturated fats. Imbalanced fat consumption with either a heavy focus on saturated and heated vegetable oils is what creates unhealthy bodies. Researchers have only recently discovered and announced inflammation as a possible cause of heart and vascular disease. Personally, I believe the leading cause of inflammation is sugar. After studying fats for over 30 years, I do believe that red meat obviously is a factor, and the primary dietary fat culprit. However, unlike those in conventional medicine who blame cholesterol as the primary cause. I believe cholesterol is merely an unwilling accomplice found at the site of the inflammation, trying to stop the whole event in the first place! Cholesterol is being instructed by the brain to be present at the inflamed site by the self-preserving nature of the human body in order to put the fire out. Cells have the ability to make cholesterol. **Over the years of seeing patients, thousands (and it is getting worse) show up at my door step with symptoms of the inability to make natural cortisone which subdues the fire of inflammation.** I realize the public is confused as to what to do.

When I first came to see Dr. Bob I had joint pain and a loss of mobility in my left femoral joint. I was also taking anti-depressants, birth control and muscle relaxants. Following Dr. Bob's advice I have greatly decreased my sugar intake. I consume little or no sodas, ice cream, candy, cakes and I avoid fast food restaurants. Eliminating sugar and processed foods while switching to organic foods as well as eating a beet daily has been difficult. However, since making these lifestyle changes I am no longer on medications and I no longer suffer with PMS, depression or muscle spasms. I also have increased mobility. I am so grateful for the treatment I have received. I am hopeful that I will keep my health and mobility while preventing any chronic illnesses.

~Dody Cuson

When the body is short on raw materials as a result of stress, sugar, toxicity, burnout, etc., it cries out to the CEO, your brain, "HELP! I need more raw materials for the adrenal glands to make enough cortisone from cholesterol to put the fires out! Have the cells make more cholesterol so I can save this person's life."

The typical patient will show up at the physician's office with high cholesterol (which is used to make cortisone), fatigue (from adrenal burnout) and pain and be told they need cholesterol lowering meds. That is like shooting the firemen! Those meds do not get to the cause of inflammation. I know that is a very simple story, but as I see it, it's the truth and nothing but the truth.

The gland maintaining and controlling cortisone is a small walnut shaped mass of high powered tissue called the adrenal gland. It is located on top of the kidney. Adrenal fatigue is poorly understood, an epidemic, and out of control in America. It can be assumed to be caused by stress and poor diet. Common body signals include bright lights irritating the eyes, craving salt and salty foods, dizziness occurring from a sitting to standing position, and the back "going-out" easily.

Adrenal fatigue can be more objectively monitored by taking your blood pressure lying down or recumbent, then standing up. Blood pressure normally should elevate from the down to up position. Adrenal activity can be monitored with mineral tissue analysis, saliva, and serum evaluation. I suggest lifestyle modification to my patients including the elimination of non-essential commitments, reducing refined sugar in breads, pastries, cookies, pastas, etc. They are told to focus on whole foods, mild exercise and I recommend an adrenal fatigue supplement protocol (see Additional Resources page for further information).

Patients need to avoid the real culprit, sugar, which has so deeply permeated our food chain, and then cholesterol levels will reset themselves naturally over time as the inflammation subsides in the body.

The scientific community has been telling the duped masses to stop eating cholesterol — No eggs, No meat, No cheese, No, No, No — for forty years. Guess what? Cholesterol levels are still high, some even with drugs. This is because your body, the self-preserving organism that it is, knows if you are stressed from eating sugar and in toxic burnout, you need cholesterol or you will die. In addition, patients need to avoid the real culprit, sugar, which has so deeply permeated our food chain, and then cholesterol levels will reset themselves naturally over time as the inflammation subsides in the body. **This may take some time in individuals with chemically poisoned livers caused by cholesterol lowering drugs that have caused some liver damage.**

A long time acquaintance of mine in his fifties, thin, non-smoker, happily married, work stressed father of three, always had elevated cholesterol. He would regularly tell me all the remedies he was taking to keep his cholesterol low. He had been prescribed a series of various cholesterol lowering drugs over the years. After he conversed with some of my patients who have seen success, he decided to give Dr. Bob a try. I laid it out for him. I told him, as I am telling you: No Sugar! Sugar is poison. It is elevating your cholesterol!! I'll never forget when he asked if he could have an egg. His lip quivered; he had not let an egg touch his lips for twenty years. Needless to say, he changed his diet from eating low-fat and high carb to consuming flax oil, complex carbs, lean meat, even some red meat, and you know the rest of the story. His cholesterol, and at no extra charge his triglycerides as well, stabilized. You can do this too.

I had high cholesterol, especially high LDL's, a slumping posture, and didn't eat enough protein foods when I first came to see Dr. DeMaria. I took Niacin daily along with aspirin and garlic to try and control the high LDL's. Dr. Bob shared that I needed to reduce my carb intake and begin eating more protein (this was difficult for me since I was accustomed to eating mostly carbs). I began eating a lower carb diet and added protein, i.e., eggs and red meat. I love that I get to eat eggs again while my cholesterol stays low!
~**Pat Dobson**

Summary

- **Fat molecules** are held together by bonds.

- **Single bonds** are saturated — solid, hard.

- **Double bonds** are unsaturated — liquid, soft.

- **Unsaturated/polyunsaturated plant sourced fats** do not have cholesterol.

- **Cis Fat** naturally fits in a cell membrane.

- **Trans fat** alters cell membrane structure.

- **Inflammation** triggers the alarm to increase cholesterol production by the cells to supply the adrenal gland cortisone building blocks.

- **Sugar and stress** are the leading causes of inflammation.

4

Fat Facts

This chapter is, by far, one of the most important pieces of information you will ever read. I promise it will be really simple. Let me set the tone. I treat patients, naturally, every day. I am not force-fed information by pharmaceutical detail men. I study the results I see with patients and use it to create more effective treatment protocols. Regardless of who you are, physiology is physiology. Water freezes at thirty-two degrees Fahrenheit no matter what your healthcare background is. The word doctor, from its Greek origin, can be translated to "teacher." My intent is to teach you about fat — not to impress you with big words, formulas or jargon. I am going to relay to you what I have seen over thirty years. This is not a blind study, money driven or hypothetical information, but observations of results, victories and setbacks from real people, the people who wake up in the morning and are hungry, have kids to feed, groceries to buy, schedules to keep, and lifestyles to maintain. So let's get to it.

I recently was having a discussion with a friend of mine about health. He lifts weights, exercises aerobically, sees natural doctors and generally, from the outside, appears to be in excellent shape for his age. I asked him the same question I am going to ask you: Do you know what trans fat is? A glassy, blank stare with a statue-like facial expression appeared as he said, "I do not have a clue what you're talking about." I questioned whether he was sure. Embarrassingly and not wanting to hurt my feelings, he responded, "No, and probably very few other people I know do either." End of conversation.

The very next day I was scheduled to speak to a group of over one hundred and thirty people about ADHD, Alzheimer's and depression. I thought, WOW! This was a mixed-age group, with various cross-cultural, socio-economic diverse attendees. I'll ask them the same question I posed to my friend. I explained to them about my research for this book and wanted a show of hands as to how many knew what trans fat was. Only ten people raised their hands. I was taken back. It occurred to me that we are truly sharing the same mindset that people had four or five hundred years ago concerning scurvy. No one knew a lack of vitamin C was killing their families, just as these individuals did not realize trans fat is the leading factor for ADHD, Alzheimer's and depression. All are in an epidemic growth pattern and no one seems to understand why. Now for the rest of the story.

Your body uses fat for fuel, insulation, to make hormones and send messages on cell membranes. It is also used to isolate toxins and provide a protective coat in blood vessels to keep them from damage and relieve pain.

For some, like my fitness trainer's husband, the thought of fat passing their lips can create convulsive gyrations. Fat gives taste to food; your body needs fat to function. This is sometimes a surprise to people. Your body uses fat for fuel, insulation, to make hormones and send messages on cell membranes. It is also used to isolate toxins and provide a protective coat in blood vessels to keep them from damage and to relieve pain.

My first easy-to-understand discussion is about a fat classification called essential fats. You see, the mass confusion about fats lays in all the classifications and possibilities. This will be easy, easy, easy.

There are two essential fats. They are termed essential because the body doesn't produce them; you need to eat them. If you don't eat them, you can't use them. These fats are used to make other fats essential for life. **My study points to a lack of quality-sourced essential fats that cause our modern health problems.** As a result, it is necessary to explain the two essential fats.

Linoleic Acid

The first essential fat I would like to introduce is called Linoleic Acid which is pronounced like it looks, lynn-o-lay-ik. Examples of the natural sources for linoleic acid include most seeds, nuts, safflower oil and sunflower oil. These fats can be eaten in oil form, and also, they are commonly found in foods as well. These food items and oils can be considered precursors. The linoleic foods you eat need to go through steps to become other important factors your body needs. These steps require vitamins and minerals such as calcium, magnesium, zinc, Vitamin B and vitamin B6 (see chart #1). Deficiencies in any of these vitamins and minerals can interrupt your body's ability to build and repair itself. I have said it before: the body is a self-healing organism. Certain enzymes are also part of the process. They can become deficient because of age and medications taken. Time for a slow breath. Reread this paragraph. What I am going to say in the next section is big.

PG1 takes away pain, makes blood cells less sticky and vessel walls more pliable. Simply put, they are heart healthy and pain relieving.

The process for linoleic acid continues on to become a final item I want to discuss next called prostaglandin one, PG1. Prostaglandins are fat, tissue-like hormones that are necessary for critical life enhancing functions. PG1 takes away pain, makes blood cells less sticky and vessel walls more pliable. Simply put, they are heart healthy and pain relieving.

There are multiple enzymes needed to complete the process. An enzyme acts as a catalyst or little freight ship moving cargo in and out of the harbor or cells. There is an enzyme called cycloxygenase. (see chart #2) This enzyme has been the target of modern pain relieving pharmaceutical research teams. Commonly called a cox inhibitor, it is the family of enzymes targeted by Vioxx and Celebrex in the formation of prostaglandin 2, PG2, which creates pain and causes blood cells to stick. When these enzymes are targeted

Chart #1

Omega-6
fatty acids

Precursor Oils

Corn, Sunflower,
Safflower & Other
Vegetable Oils
(from snack foods)

▽

Linoleic Acid

▽

B6, Zinc, Mg, D-6-D

TransFats & ★
Hydrogenated Fats
"French Fries"
FOOD ADDITIVES
Inhibit The Process

▽

Gamma-
linolenic Acid

▽

Dihomo-gamma-
llinolenic Acid **Can Make Arachidonic Acid** ➤ See Chart #2

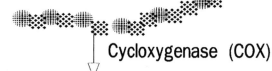

Cycloxygenase (COX)

▽

Prostaglandin #1

Pain **Relieving**

Chart #2

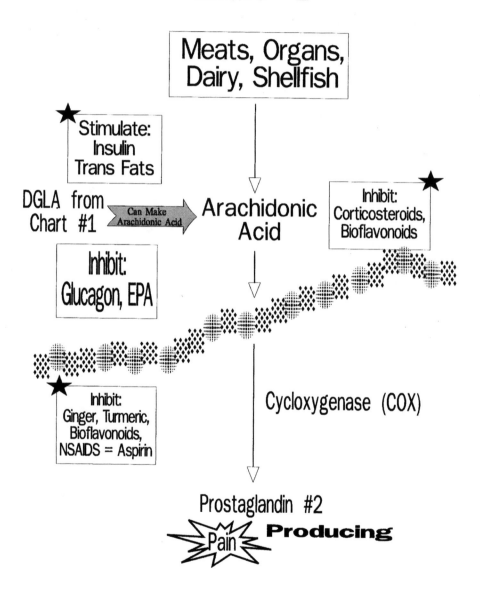

Meats, Organs, Dairy, Shellfish

★ Stimulate:
Insulin
Trans Fats

DGLA from Chart #1 — Can Make Arachidonic Acid → Arachidonic Acid

Inhibit:
Corticosteroids,
Bioflavonoids ★

Inhibit:
Glucagon, EPA

★ Inhibit:
Ginger, Turmeric,
Bioflavonoids,
NSAIDS = Aspirin

Cycloxygenase (COX)

Prostaglandin #2

Pain Producing

for one function, the ripple effect creates physiologic havoc elsewhere. You will read more about cox inhibitors in Chapter 10.

PG2 is necessary so you feel pain and don't bleed to death, and therefore, understand you need rest and healing.

I got ahead of myself with PG2. We now need to back up a bit. Linoleic acid in its passage can also become another fat called arachidonic acid. Arachidonic acid can become PG2. PG2 is necessary so you feel pain and don't bleed to death, and therefore, understand you need rest and healing. The interim step creating arachidonic acid is in the chart. The fat name is called, *dihomogamma linolenic acid*, D-GLA. Your body in its ability to self-regulate needs to increase the formation of arachidonic acid for balance of other fats. The creation of arachidonic acid is one of the reasons some scientists believe we need to eat less food, fat, and oil with linoleic acid features. We get too much linoleic acid eating snack foods with safflower and sunflower oil. Avoiding trans fat is important, but replacing it with an excess of these two oils, which becomes D-GLA, causes pain, sticky blood cells, weak vascular walls and is not the best option either.

The critical point to the whole process which is not widely known is the fact that **the man-made, heated vegetable oil**

Man-made, heated vegetable oil processing, called hydrogenation, creates trans fat.

processing, called hydrogenation, creates trans fat which also derails the process (see chapter 8). Not only does trans fat derail the process, but its bad effects last for a long time.

Do you remember in science class when your teacher talked about Madame Curie's discovery of the half-life of uranium? Well, trans fat has a half life as well. Through research and experience, I have learned that the half-life of trans fat is fifty-one days. That may or may not seem like a lot, but understand how half-life works. When you eat a bag of chips, a deep fried doughnut, cream-filled cookies or anything with hydrogenated fat, it takes your body 51 days to properly metabolize and eliminate HALF of it. In another 51 days, HALF of that, 25 percent, is still in your body. That's 102 days, over 3 months, and you still haven't processed all of the trans fat you just ate!! If you are eating trans fat every day — and you are if you eat snack foods, prepackaged foods and deep fried foods — imagine how much trans fat is congesting your body from years of this eating pattern. That's a pretty nauseating thought. Take two deep breaths and read this again.

Now you can call your old college roommate and tell him you know why little Joey has ADHD, or why you have depression and are not responding to medication, or your auntie has Alzheimer's and is failing quickly (all are precipitated by trans fat; see Dr. Bob's Guide to Stop ADHD in 18 Days, Chapter 11). Now do you see how big this really is?! Researchers in haste, ignorance and greed, have most people believing margarine is better than butter. Do you remember my show of hands? **No one, in all reality at this time, knows that what they are eating is actually silently and slowly killing them.** Let's continue; hang in there!

I need to make a couple of real life clinical comments. This will require you to be honest with how your body feels, and in fact may be a revelation for many. What I need to add to your understanding is that arachidonic acid with its negative results can be directly sourced with no processing from dairy, red meat, mollusks, and shell fish. These particular items can directly become arachidonic acid and processed to PG2. Clinically, I strongly encourage my patients to be conscious of dairy consumption and pain. Yes, you read right. The white mustache dairy campaign promotes aches, pain, and limited motion in the body.

**Yes, you read right.
The white mustache dairy campaign
promotes aches, pain, and limited motion in the body.**

This direct sourcing of arachidonic acid which makes PG2, the pain-causing prostaglandin, can be accelerated by trans fat consumption, insulin, alcohol, food coloring and preservatives (see Chart #2). The same process is inhibited by cortisone, bioflavinoids, turmeric in mustard, boswella (an herb), and aspirin. Now you can see why what you eat has a direct impact on how you feel. The reason you are to eat your five servings of fruits and vegetables is to promote pain relief and control PG2. Eating your basic fast-food meal depletes vitamins and minerals, sabotaging PG1 and inviting pain into your body. I require all of my patients to keep track in a journal what they eat so they can see what they are putting into their bodies and what could be the causes of pain. **I empower them with information with which they can be proactive contributors to a healthy lifestyle.**

The reason you are to eat your five servings of fruits and vegetables is to promote pain relief and control PG2.

Their responses to my recommendations and protocols are directly affected by their choices. **Some make the changes and experience a higher quality of life while others stay in denial and subsequently continue to suffer.** It is always interesting after special holidays or on Mondays after big weekends of bad eating. My patients are experiencing pain, rationalizing their "small" piece of pie or "little" cookie as they indicate portion size with hand gestures on the small but lethal quantity of dietary "deviation" they imposed on their bodies.

It is time to move on to the other essential fat. We are not completely finished with linoleic acid, but I will bring it all together at the end of the next section.

Summary of Linoleic Acid — PG1 and PG2

- ➤ It is essential for life and must be consumed.

- ➤ It is used to create and support bodily functions for optimal health.

- ➤ It requires calcium, magnesium, zinc, enzymes, quality-sourced, whole food B vitamins and B6 to evolve to PG1 or to arachidonic acid and PG2.

- ➤ It develops into pain relieving, non-blood cell sticking PG1 or if consumed too liberally, causes PG2 and pain and sticky blood cells.

- ➤ Its metabolic steps are **detoured** by sugar, alcohol, insulin, aspirin, food additives, minerals, and enzymes.

- ➤ Its metabolic steps are **sabotaged** by trans fat intake.

- ➤ There is evidence-based experience from evaluations of diet journals that linoleic acid is adequately consumed in the current American daily diet pattern.

- ➤ It is sourced from most nuts, seeds, safflower and sunflower oils.

Alpha-Linolenic Acid

Alpha-Linolenic acid, ALA, is the second essential fatty acid. The activity of ALA is comparable to its counter part linoleic acid with a few exceptions. First, ALA is not normally consumed in the typical American diet. It requires a metabolic pathway that starts with items including flaxseeds, mixed greens, greens, and walnuts among other foods. These precursor foods need to go through steps with quality sourced ingredients including enzymes, calcium, magnesium, zinc, whole food B vitamins and B6, like linoleic acid requires (see chart 3). The process can be inhibited by insulin, alcohol, food additives, vitamin, mineral and enzyme deficiencies precipitated by anti-nutrients like sugar and stress. Trans fat sabotages the metabolic process as it does for linoleic acid.

ALA continues on to be several very important long chained fats needed for heart and brain/nerve health. The first is *eicosapentaenoic acid*, EPA. EPA is the fat you will see being suggested for heart smart people. It can be directly sourced from marine sources or the ALA pathway. The other long chain fat is called *docosahexaenoic acid*, DHA. DHA is needed for proper brain and nervous system function. My research with a group of participants in a study that I designed and monitored overwhelmingly suggested that the breakdown of DHA through the ALA pathway precipitated by trans fat consumption was the primary cause of ADHD, ADD, and hyperactivity (see *Dr. Bob's Guide to Stop ADHD, ADD, and Hyperactivity in 18 Days*, Chapter 18 available through Drugless Healthcare Solutions at www.druglesscare.com). ALA progresses on to become another prostaglandin or fat tissue hormone, prostaglandin 3, PG3, which is a pain relieving, non-sticking blood cell prostaglandin.

Controversy over fat metabolism is common.

Controversy over fat metabolism is common. I would like to express my observations gathered from real people, with actual life issues, not experimental lab animals or controlled human research environments.

Pain must be managed through lifestyle changes, specifically through eating foods to enhance health.

As I have mentioned previously, taking cox inhibitors, aspirin and the like does not correct the problem but only hides the symptoms. These items are tolerable. Pain must be managed through lifestyle changes, specifically through eating foods to enhance health.

In my experience, I have seen and treated the devastation of kidney and liver disease caused by pain medication prescribed by a physician with the instructions to take it "like candy." I have seen organ transplants as a result of pain medication stressing the system. Cortisone, prednisone and other steroids over time, can be disfiguring. I recommend organic-sourced, high-lignan omega processed flax oil or gel capsules to my patients and I see consistent, long-term results.

I recommend organic-sourced, high-lignan omega processed flax oil or gel capsules to my patients and I see consistent, long-term results.

The public is encouraged to consume marine life for sources of EPA and DHA. Diet logs suggest we consume similar levels of marine products today as we did in the 1970s. I do not believe more deep water fish is the answer. The reason you will read about salmon and salmon capsules for a heart and brain source of EPA and DHA is because nearly all researchers believe the body is not genetically capable of making enough of these long chained fats. Taking salmon capsules as a consistent fat supplement may in fact thin your blood too much resulting in a stroke or internal bleeding. I would suggest having your bleeding time checked. I would not — I will repeat myself — I would not take flax or salmon capsules while you are taking blood thinners without being monitored by your healthcare provider.

Here is a question for you. Why did we have a human body that worked 30, 40, or 50 years ago and it is now not making enough EPA and DHA? There are two answers. One, trans fat

The source of minerals, vitamins and enzymes in our environment is so pitifully low that Americans are mineral and vitamin deficient.

sabotages your body's ability to make EPA and DHA from up to 51 days continuing for 102 days. Secondly, the source of minerals, vitamins and enzymes in our environment is so pitifully low that Americans are mineral and vitamin deficient. Vitamins, minerals and enzymes are also needed to have success in the ALA process. "But I take my One-A-Day A to Z tablet packed with everything I need!" you exclaim. However, what I know and what other natural practitioners know is that these vitamins are usually synthetic. They are processed, isolated and fractionalized. They are chemical compounds created in a lab and they do not always fit into the cell structure of the body. I can tell you this with confidence because I see real people everyday who bring me their boxes, bags, and plastic containers of mega ballistic vitamins and still feel lousy. Generally, low-dosage, cold-processed, food-sourced products are best. **If you take supplements and you're not progressing, you may want to contemplate making some modifications.** In my practice, I use whole food based supplements that have not been isolated and fractionalized to large or small sizes.

We have epidemic sickness in advanced Western cultures because we have over-processed foods, including vitamins and mineral supplements, making them less effective.

Even with all the technology available today, there are particles not yet discovered in whole foods that are required for life. We have epidemic sickness in advanced Western cultures because we have over-processed foods, including vitamins and mineral supplements, making them less effective. Natural function is based on low-dose levels. The ALA pathway requires the right ingredients to function.

One consolation is synthetic vitamins, especially the larger ones, make awesome slingshot ammunition. They leave a mark when you hit the target. Go on have some fun! Get a sling shot and practice hitting your empty bottles.

Aspirin is consumed by the billions. I am totally aware of that. Hormone replacement therapy was taken by the millions — people died. Cox inhibitors (see Chapter 10) for pain relief destroyed thousands in its short but profitable life. Millions of dollars were spent by direct marketing to promote Vioxx use. Doctors and patients appeared to have the mind set that new is better. Be aware. Aspirin works by inhibiting the formation of PG2, the pain causing prostaglandin, resulting in pain relief, not healing. Aspirin also interferes with the formation of PG1 and PG3. I have made information available to you. With your patience, study, and perseverance you can create a pain-free life and emotional state once again.

Summary of Alpha-Linolenic Acid

➢ It is one of the essential fats you must consume.

➢ It is sourced indirectly from flax, mixed greens, green foods, and selected nuts and seeds.

➢ It evolves to EPA for heart health and DHA for brain and nervous system function.

➢ It is processed to become prostaglandin 3 which is pain relieving and non-blood cell sticking.

➢ It requires calcium, magnesium, zinc, B vitamins, B6, and enzymes to process.

➢ It is inhibited by insulin, food additives, alcohol enzymes, vitamin and mineral deficiencies, aspirin, and cox inhibitors.

➢ Analysis of diet journals indicate that ALA is lacking from the standard American diet.

➢ It is sabotaged by trans fat.

Summary of Non-Essential Arachidonic Acid

- ➤ It can be created from processing linoleic acid.

- ➤ It is directly sourced from the diet through dairy, meat, mollusk and shell fish consumption.

- ➤ It can evolve to PG2 which is pain creating and blood cell adhering.

- ➤ PG2 formation is inhibited by aspirin, cox inhibitors, bioflavinoids, vitamin C, cortisone, selected fat, turmeric and boswella.

- ➤ PG2 formation is accelerated by trans fat, insulin, alcohol, food additives.

One last thought before I move on. This will be a shocker to the research scientist in the pharmaceutical industry knowing that the public has access to this information. **Taking aspirin, physiologically, is a temporary band-aid for a deeper problem.** The aspirin makers generate billions of dollars and are aware that aspirin is media driven and not the answer for everyone. That is why we have the cox inhibitors and other pain relieving options for the 80 percent of Americans who live in chronic pain. Aspirin does not promote natural function in the human body. It is wrong. Now, that doesn't mean to throw out all your aspirin. You will need to modify your diet to achieve optimal health by removing refined sugar and trans fat from your diet and by limiting dairy, red meat, and alcohol. Can you do it? Yes, you can! Knowledge is power. Have your prothrombin time, your bleeding time, checked. Aspirin side effects may be causing some of your below par bodily functions which you or your physician have not connected. Aspirin slows bone fracture healing. A thought — is it a factor in osteoporosis?

Aspirin does not promote natural function in the human body. It is wrong.

Did you ever stop to wonder why we did not have problems like this before? Could it be trans fat? Overeating sugar? Both are found in nearly every item in a conventional grocery store and franchise fast foods restaurant. **The frustration for most patients I see today is the fear of getting a heart attack, stroke, or some other vascular problem.** Pharmaceutical driven healthcare providers do what they are told. I know this is a bold statement, but information is out there for them to learn and is a part of their studies, but it is falling on deaf ears.

The patients who seek natural drugless care are capable of achieving a pain-free lifestyle without the side effects of prescription or over-the-counter medication.

Pain relief driven treatment programs create massive revenues in our medical mindset economy. The patients who seek natural drugless care are capable of achieving a pain-free lifestyle without the side effects of prescription or over-the-counter medication.

≈

End Notes

NUTRITION ACTION HEALTHLETTER, December 2002.

5

Omega Fat: Tying the Essential Fats Together

I have mentioned that the confusion in fats can lay in all the classifications, chains, formulas, bonds and chemical groups. We are now going to turn it up a notch. This is one classification you want to know about so when you talk about trans fat, you'll present yourself well.

The two essential fats that we described previously can be further separated in name and structure because of the double bond position. Double bonds can occur between any two carbons in a carbon chain. Plants insert double bonds at different points in fatty acid chains than animals. This affects properties and the effects of the fats. There is a named position in the chain determined by the location in the molecule. This, in turn, determines the placement of the double bond in its relation to the methyl end (end of the fat chain). A double bond placed three places from the methyl end is called an Omega-3 fat. This is also known as an alpha-linolenic acid, an essential fat. A common precursor would be flax oil. Omega-3 fat will be in the media for years to come. Not commonly understood by the public, omega-3 fat is a part of EPA, DHA and PG3 (see Chart #3, page 42).

Chart #3

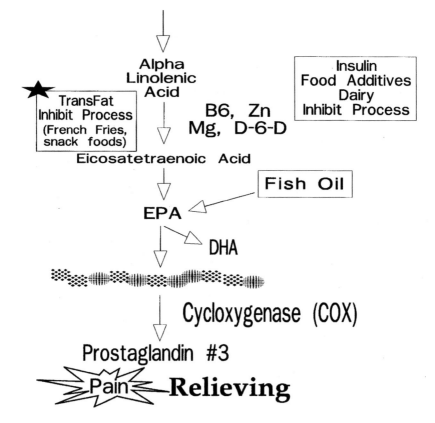

Omega-3
fatty acids

Precursor Oils

Flax Oil,
Leafy Greens
Walnuts, Grasses

Alpha
Linolenic
Acid

★ TransFat
Inhibit Process
(French Fries,
snack foods)

Insulin
Food Additives
Dairy
Inhibit Process

B6, Zn
Mg, D-6-D

Eicosatetraenoic Acid

Fish Oil

EPA

DHA

Cycloxygenase (COX)

Prostaglandin #3

Pain—Relieving

There is one more omega location to be discussed. When a double bond placement is six positions from the methyl end it is called an omega-6 fat. It also is an essential fat and is found in safflower, sunflower, walnut and sesame oils. The precursor name is linoleic acid. It can be metabolized to PG1 and PG2. Omega-6 fats are commonly found in snack foods. You will see these oils, called expeller-pressed, in the labeling process to replace trans fat (see Chart #1, page 28).

The omega position may create confusion in your understanding of the terminology. I remember Omega-3 is from flax and fish like salmon. Omega-3 is also known as DHA and EPA. You will read more about these over time. My evidenced based research suggests that flax, greens, walnuts, with additional supplementation of whole food vitamins and minerals is what your body needs. Once again, trans fat and sugar inhibit your body's absorption and utilization of what it requires. But also omega-6 fats can slow, stop, and even destroy omega-3 fat production. Over time, with the trans fat media hype, most of the snack food manufacturers will focus on omega-6 fats — especially the oleic versions — which can be heated They may come up with other sources, like esterified oil. For your own sake, if you want to eat items with safflower, sunflower or any other oil, go ahead and do it. But, take a tip from Dr. Bob — make sure you are taking your flax oil, eating your greens, taking your vitamins and minerals, and avoid raising insulin with sugar. Of course, no trans fat! Focus on whole foods after you deviate. If you start getting pain, hormonal or emotional distress, (see Chapter 10) you are probably overdoing the omega-6 fats.

Make sure you are taking your flax oil, eating your greens, taking your vitamins and minerals, and avoid raising insulin with sugar. Of course, no trans fat

Never Too Late

Want to stick around to see your great-grandchildren? In a study of more than 2,300 people in 11 European countries, those who ate a healthy Mediterranean diet, exercised, didn't smoke, and drank alcohol moderately were less likely to die in their 70s and 80s.

The researchers gave the highest diet scores to people who ate less meat, dairy, and saturated fat and more fruits, vegetables, beans, fish, grains, nuts, and unsaturated fats. People with the highest scores had a 23 percent lower risk of dying during the 10-year study.

Not smoking and staying physically active each cut the risk about 35 percent. People who drank alcohol moderately had a 22 percent lower risk. And the folks who scored high on all four measures were 65 percent less likely to die of any cause, including heart disease and cancer.

What to do: All of the above. Just don't equate a Mediterranean diet with pizza or lasagna. And don't use the study as an excuse to start drinking.

J. Amer. Med. Assoc. 292: 292: 1433, 2004

6

Fat Phobia

In the realm of the diet conscious, the 1990s could easily be categorized as an age of fat phobia. Fear of fats. You think if you eat any kind of fat you will gain weight. People across America started reading food labels, not for nutritional quality, but for fat quantity. We bought foods with the least amount of fat possible, purchased the leanest cuts of meats, and ate salad without dressing. Not exactly tasty. I can remember friends eating boxes of Entenmanns's Fat-Free Brownie cookies rationalizing all the sugar and fillers with no fat. And then there were fat free potato chips. **I know people who, excited about being able to eat junk food and not get fat, would eat until full only to have the chips literally "go right through them."** Was it worth it? I doubt it. In this chapter you will learn the importance of NOT avoiding the right kind of fat.

We have more technology and ongoing research at this moment of time versus any other period in recorded history. The research is often funded by a segment of industry attempting to take a new product to the market place. I am all for the free enterprise system. Competition is good — it creates a better "mouse trap." My frustration with science today is who is telling the truth and who is pulling the wool over society's eyes. It was recently reported in the media that all but one of the physician-scientists suggesting lower cholesterol levels were on the payroll of an industry positioned to reap huge profits by their recommendations

> **My frustration with science today is who is telling the truth and who is pulling the wool over society's eyes.**

(AP, 2004). The cholesterol lowering industry is a mega-billion dollar conglomerate. Paradoxically, the statin drugs discussed in the article mask the real cause of high cholesterol and complicate the situation by precipitating liver disease.

Man's continuous desire to learn more, at the expense of fooling Mother Nature, started in 1873. Heat was added to vegetable oil with the help of a catalyst, an element that forces change. The product of the experiment is what we today refer to as hydrogenated fat, trans fat, or more recently, partially hydrogenated fat. **These are man-made compounds sourced from vegetable oils.** To simplify my discussion and your understanding, I will use the term **trans fat** in reference to hydrogenated or partially hydrogenated fats. Today, these trans fats have permeated nearly every level of food source taken in by the unsuspecting, uninformed consumer. This is a multi-tiered dilemma. It affects a very broad, global part of our economy. Originally thought to be health promoting, the actual fact is, trans fat has become the cause of health problems. This is the foundational fact for the entire book. Trans fat interferes with the body's ability to take the food you eat, like beans, lettuce, nuts, etc., to its final destination, including steps to reduce pain, promote brain, cardiovascular and hormone health, and a long list of bodily functions.

> **Trans fat interferes with the body's ability to take the food you eat, like beans, lettuce, nuts, etc., to its final destination, including steps to reduce pain, promote brain, cardiovascular and hormone health, and a long list of bodily functions.**

The butter-promoting dairy association was successful in limiting the exposure and utilization of trans fat in the early 1900s. WWII created a demand for an alternative to butter to be used by the masses. The patriotic American public wanting to support the cause readily consumed the new "oleo margarine" so the soldiers in the trenches could have real butter.

Retracing my life to my younger years, I remember having a package of semi-clear "goop" with a red button that contained, I would suspect, yellow dye. I always enjoyed the snap and pop, then the squeeze, magically watching the container become mysteriously yellow with every squeeze. The real benefit? This mixture was great for camping and vacationers on the go. As time went on, the name evolved to "margarine." It did not need to be refrigerated because it would not spoil. I guess knowing that fact, we all should have known better. If a product does not decompose, it probably should not be eaten. The rules do not change. I encourage my patients not to eat food that does not break down and return to the ecosystem to be used again.

> **If a product does not decompose, it probably should not be eaten.**

Do you remember some of those original margarine commercials and advertisements convincing us about the benefit of convenient margarine, whipped and easy to spread? One brand was so bold as to show Mother Nature being fooled. How elementary. But it worked and people today, even some of you reading these words, would be mortified to let butter pass your lips. I recently had one patient who watched his diet strictly for over twenty years, never letting a tiny morsel of butter or egg into his body because of his continually and unmoving high cholesterol. He celebrated with me because his cholesterol finally plummeted while eating eggs and butter as a part of his diversified lifestyle modification.

The fast food industry was gladly pressured into switching from perishable, expensive lard and beef tallow to easy to store, long shelf-life vegetable oils which were partially or totally hydrogenated.

My clinical awareness of fat phobia and fat confusion started at the same time as the fast food switch. I was not raised on fast food. I would have to believe most baby boomers ate most dinner meals at home. Our families were not stretched with moms' working and forty-two activities for all the kids.

Today, there are fewer children at home, but the activities start from birth with the current generations taking babies three months old and younger to the day care center. All the activity, distractions and no time created a demand for a cheap, fast, tasty and easy-to-make line of meals. Out of nowhere the multi-zillion dollar a year processed food industry started and flourished world wide. Everybody was happy. All the dilemmas were temporarily resolved until we started getting fat and sick. No one knew who to blame, and quite frankly, we still are arguing into this new millennium.

Physiology does not change. Food is measured in units of energy called calories. One gram of protein creates four units or calories. Carbohydrates also create four units of energy per one gram. Fat, on the other hand, creates nine grams of energy. You can flip this around and say you get four or nine grams of potential weight gain for every gram of whatever you choose to eat. Now I have simplified a massive problem here. There is a web of possibilities that alter this formula. For the purpose of this discussion people were getting fat. What was the cause?

Not Just Low-Fat

A low-fat diet that's rich in vegetables, beans and whole grains lowers LDL ("bad") cholesterol more than an equally low-fat diet without those extras.

Researchers supplied 120 adults who had high cholesterol with one of two diets. Both were low in fat (30 percent of calories) and saturated fat (10 percent of calories).

However, the *ordinary* low-fat diet included no whole grains or soy, only five daily servings of fruits and vegetables, and lots of prepared foods (like lower-fat versions of cheese, snack foods and frozen lasagna).

After four weeks, LDL dropped more (14 points) on the low-fat plus diet than on the ordinary low-fat diet (7 points).

What to do: It's not clear whether the fiber (40 grams a day), soy (16 grams per 2,000 calories), garlic (1½ cloves a day) or other components of the low-fat plus diet accounted for its impact on cholesterol. Either way, it makes sense to eat more vegetables, beans and whole grains.

Annals of Internal Medicine 142, 725, 793, 2005

Remember, everyone has been thoroughly convinced the cause of heart disease was high fat and high cholesterol consumed in our diets. That is why the fast food industry flipped to vegetable oil with **no cholesterol** while **no fat, low fat** drove the food marketing starting in the nineteen seventies. However, the public is fatter than ever and cardiovascular disease continues to be the leading cause of death in America. We have added more fat-related disease conditions all tied with improper fat metabolism disrupted by trans fat — including Alzheimer's, emotional distress, pain syndromes, cancers, and chronic degenerative health. **The latter issues have not been connected to each other by the conventional medical thinkers. It is only recently that trans fat was discovered to be unhealthy by research scientists. The masses have been persuaded that cholesterol is the poison.**

> **We have added more fat-related disease conditions all tied with improper fat metabolism disrupted by trans fat — including Alzheimer's, emotional distress, pain syndromes, cancers, and chronic degenerative health.**

Evidence-based patient monitoring by myself and other natural health care providers suggests that through diet journaling, examinations and tissue analysis the "low-fat, highly-refined, carbohydrate diet" and pharmaceutical medications assault on the body are not working. Someone has missed the target. **People are dying as a technologically-based system remains out of touch with reality and looks the other way, focusing on making more money at the expense of human life. That is a bold but true statement, to say the least.**

What are some of the common health problems for Americans despite 10-15 years of consuming low-fat foods? The answer is clogged arteries and heart disease. Here's why:

1. The medical media has infused in us that a diet low in fat is best. Fully eight percent of school children now think that the healthiest diet is one that eliminates *all fat* — a death sentence diet.

2. Studies prove that eating less fat causes the body to make more fat at a dramatically increased rate, which is then stored more easily. So eating low fat will cause more fat. And, unlike the clinical studies proving this fact, there is no proof at all that eating a high-fat diet causes obesity.

> **Studies prove that eating less fat causes the body to make more fat at a dramatically increased rate.**

3. Oxidation, cell breakdown, of fats can cause cancer. Saturated fats, like meat and dairy, do not oxidize easily. Fully 41 percent of all physicians polled were under the mistaken belief that saturated fats were the oxidation culprits in cancer. The fact is fake fats and low-fat concoctions are the real culprits: just read the ingredients on a can of Pringles.

4. Along with an Omega-3 fat supplement like a tablespoon of raw flax oil for two to three years, consumption of monounsaturated fat like olive oil must also be part of the diet. That's why I recommend extra-virgin, first-pressed olive oil for salad dressings, food preparation, and cooking. If oxidation of fats acts like *rusting* in your body, olive oil is Rustoleum.

> **If oxidation of fats acts like *rusting* in your body, olive oil is Rustoleum.**

5. Low-fat diets are dramatically low in vitamins A, D, E, F, and K, the very nutrients you need to maintain a healthy heart and circulatory system. Conversely, low-fat diets lack the fat necessary for your body to absorb many of the nutrients from fruits and vegetables.

6. Almost no one can persist on a diet of 20 percent fat. Depression sets in; life becomes a bore and social well-being is distorted. The Mediterranean Diet is a better diet. It offers better health, is delicious and is easy to stick with.

7. The Zone Diet, Sugar-Busters, Atkins, Ornish, Pritiken and the rest all have something to offer. But the research shows that it is *a simple reduction in calories* that causes you to lose weight. While insulin is critical, the simplistic reasoning for the relationship between insulin and their diets is flawed. In fact, the Mediterranean Diet is better than all of these.

8. All the low-fat, zero-cholesterol concoctions are unhealthy products loaded with trans fats. Prefabricated meals and snacks from "food factories" are a disaster for your heart and health. The olive oil rich Mediterranean Diet contains no trans fats at all.

All the low-fat, zero-cholesterol concoctions are unhealthy products loaded with trans fats.

9. An olive oil Mediterranean Diet as consumed in Crete and Spain is even healthier than a Japanese diet. Japanese people consuming a lower-fat diet had much more heart disease than did Cretans consuming higher fat and a Mediterranean fare. While the Japanese diet has benefits over the average American diet, it is definitely not the best. In fact, the Japanese suffer from large numbers of strokes and high rates of cancer probably due to the low fat intake and low cholesterol levels.

10. Spain, the largest producer of olive oil, has the greatest life expectancy in the Western world.

11. Extreme low-fat diets of 20 percent fat, while disastrous to your health, are considered very healthy by most American physicians.

12. Eighty-two percent of polled physicians had no idea that low-fat diets *lower* HDL (high density lipids, the good fat) levels in the body.

As a result of the fat phobia, people are afraid of the one item that they need more than ever: quality and physiologically balanced oil. The information being shouted from the ranks of natural health care providers needs to permeate the schools, media, magazines and cyberspace. Quality, balanced, natural fat is your friend. This includes both vegetable and animal sources. You need fat to survive. Fats insulate the myelin sheath which surrounds our nerves allowing our brains to communicate with our bodies. Without necessary fats, there would be gaps in the message sent to our bodies and there would be no "communication." Fats are also important for our joints. They act as lubricants for movement much like engine oil lubricates gears and pistons. Besides the indicator light on the dashboard lighting up and telling you it's time for an oil change, your car may start to run rough, sputter, and emit foul fumes. Your body is no different. Without quality, balanced, natural fats, your body will start to break down and run rough. Fats lubricate your skin from the inside out. The list could go on. Every cell membrane in your body is made of fat and needs fat. **Fat phobia has paralyzed the common sense out of the public.** The **critical key** is eating **no trans fat** and consuming limited amounts of saturated fat.

There are a couple permitted oils in which to cook, **but any time you heat oil, you change the chemical structure. Eating these items consistently always results in poor health.**

Americans are pattern eaters. We eat donuts for breakfast, Danishes for a snack, fries and a burger for lunch, and sugar loaded cookies for an afternoon pick me up followed by a quick dinner with dessert and grazing before bed only to start over again. And virtually every one of these either contains or is cooked in trans fat.

All is not lost. Cutting edge food manufacturers are starting to create healthy items. Health-conscious Americans vote with their wallets. Look what is happening to the Krispy Kreme doughnut king. According to a recent financial document, Krispy Kreme's sales are dropping (E*Trade Financial, 2005). Are some consumers becoming more health savvy? It would seem so.

Now, it is time to learn about fat.

Before making Dr. DeMaria's recommended lifestyle changes I had stomach issues, mid-back tightness, lower back discomfort after physical activity and neck soreness when turning to the side. I modified my eating habits by eliminating milk, cheese and cutting down on processed foods. The education on food ingredients has helped tremendously with shopping and planning meals for myself and my family. The concept provided by Dr. DeMaria's office of good nutrition and exercise is what I believe is the future of all-around wellness.

~Lori Kotanidee

End Notes

Associated Press. *The Chronicle-Telegram*. Elyria, Ohio. October 17, 2004.

E*Trade Financial. April 29, 2005. {online}. Available: http://us.etrade.com. April 30, 2005.

7

Correcting Cholesterol Confusion

There is cholesterol and saturated fat confusion. Because of blind ignorance and fear, the greedy pharmaceutical companies take advantage of the public. **Because of the fear of high cholesterol, we have trans fat introduced in the marketplace. The food industry responded to the high cholesterol scare and introduced trans fat thinking it was a safer alternative.**

Cholesterol controlled dietary intake will not consistently lower your cholesterol.

Cholesterol is a very important steroid building block for hormones critical for healthy existence.

Cholesterol is neither bad nor good. The term LDL cholesterol and HDL cholesterol creates the misconception that cholesterol is fat. It is a special alcohol molecule called a sterol. Cholesterol controlled dietary intake will not consistently lower your cholesterol. There are other factors. It has properties that create a softening effect on blood vessels made hard by too much saturated fat. In technical terms, cholesterol makes cell membranes more fluid by inserting itself between the saturated fats in the cell membrane. Cholesterol is a very important steroid building block for hormones which are critical for healthy existence.

Lipids, as mentioned above (HDL and LDL), are made up of a collection of molecules called triglycerides which consist of three fatty acids that are attached to a three-carbon glycerol molecule. We eat triglycerides in our foods. They can also be made and stored in the body from excess carbohydrate intake which can then be measured in a blood test. The triglycerides and cholesterol portions of a blood test seem to strike a chord of fear like no other for most patients. There are three types of fatty acids that can attach to glycerol and create triglycerides, saturated, monounsaturated and polyunsaturated fatty acids.

Lipoproteins are many large particles or globules composed of fats, proteins and related compounds that contain cholesterol and carry them around in the blood. There are two for our discussion, LDL and HDL.

LDL, short for low density lipoprotein, is a globule that carries cholesterol in the blood. Cholesterol carried by LDL is sent to the vascular walls. It has been known to adhere to the wall and over time can accumulate, narrowing the vessel size and interfering with the lifeline of oxygen and nutrient **LDL cholesterol acts as a fire extinguisher.** transportation of blood. The cholesterol is being sent to prevent hardening of the vascular wall by saturated fat. LDL cholesterol is there, acting as a fire extinguisher.

HDL, short for high density lipoprotein, is also a globule that carries cholesterol in the blood. When cholesterol is in this form, it is leaving the vascular wall. HDL is considered good cholesterol because it is assumed this cholesterol is present when the blood vessels are healthy and not there narrowing the size of the blood vessel size. That is the theory that created the fat phobia and cholesterol mania in Western cultures during the 1980s. Researchers were aware that vegetable oils were not a source of cholesterol. They concluded that when people had heart attacks, it was because they ate red meat and high cholesterol or fat dense foods. They quickly, without adequate testing and investigating, determined that the little known or used properties of heated vegetable oils **without cholesterol** would be a quality viable alternative. **This was the beginning of mass production and use of trans fat, hydrogenated or partially hydrogenated fat.**

An entire massive media campaign started. Prior to the early 1970s, no one had a clue what their cholesterol level was. Though an anti cholesterol campaign to prevent heart disease has existed for decades, it has seen nominal success. However, the compensatory problems from lowering cholesterol are commonly seen today in the reproductive systems with erectile dysfunction and hormone replacement therapy. Other side-effects of commonly used cholesterol lowering drugs or statins include liver disease and the depletion of coenzyme Q10, (CO Q10). Cholesterol is lowered with statin drugs, interfering with the mechanism of cholesterol being shuffled over to do one of its secondary jobs in the sexual reproduction system and in making pain and inflammation relieving cortisone. Incidentally, one of the statin side effects is muscle pain. Take a good look at the contraindictions of Lipitor some time. It's all right there.

> **I believe cholesterol will be acquitted and sugar will be sentenced as the major accomplice along with other foods and food additives promoting inflammation.**

Time will tell, but my bet is that yes, an inflammation-causing diet consisting of too much sugar, dairy, and trans fat plays the major role in heart disease. I believe cholesterol will be acquitted and sugar will be sentenced as the major accomplice along with other foods and food additives promoting inflammation. Taking statin drugs is like shooting the firemen on the way to the fire. LDL cholesterol is being delivered intentionally as a survival move by the body. Cholesterol is there to correct damage. **Drugs that lower cholesterol interfere with the body's natural defense mechanisms.** These drugs bring in BILLIONS, yes, BILLIONS of dollars. The pharmaceutical companies have their cake and can eat it too. They have everyone duped and are laughing all the way to the bank.

Are you ready for some earth shattering news? You can actually lower your cholesterol without liver plugging drugs. Dr.

You can lower your cholesterol up to 40 percent by adding beet fiber to your diet.

Gina Nick, in her book, *Clinical Purification*, stated that through clinically proven research, you can lower your cholesterol up to 40 percent by adding beet fiber to your diet. Yes, you read correctly — beets. Cholesterol attaches itself to the fiber and is released through the colon. Oatmeal has similar properties. In addition, I encourage my patients to minimize refined sugar by using safe sugar substitutes (see Chapter 13) as they go through their transition from good, better, best. You might not like beets, I understand. I don't care for Brussels sprouts, but if someone suggested a food item that would minimize another medication with severe side effects, I would do it until I eliminated the cause of my problem. The cause of the problem — not to be redundant — is inflammation caused by refined sugar, of which the average American eats an alarming amount at an excess of 150 pounds per year, and trans fat, which was actually thought to be the hero.

Beets can be baked, steamed or pressure cooked. Do not boil them. Do not eat canned or pickled beets. Bake beets at 400° Fahrenheit for one hour. Cut them in slices about ½" to ¾" thick. Put a small amount of water in the bottom or your baking dish. Cover, and check with a fork for tenderness. Let them cool or eat them with olive or flax oil. Your stool (bowel movement) or urine may be red.

When I began care with Dr. DeMaria, I had very high cholesterol. My conventional doctor wanted to start me on Lipitor. After reading about this drug and the side effects, I decided to try something else. I have cut way back on sugar and I don't go close to vending machines — no pop or soda. I have also started the ABC's to health — apple, beets and carrots. It has been difficult reducing my sugar intake; no pies, cakes, junk food including chips, Tostitos and Doritos. Since following Dr. Bob's advice I have lowered my cholesterol some 20 points and lowered my triglycerides 170 points. I also have no aches or pains like I did before.   **~Fred Smith**

Summary

➢ **Cholesterol** is neither bad nor good .

➢ **Cholesterol** is not a fat.

➢ **Cholesterol** is needed by the body to function. If levels are lower than 160, other health problems can result.

➢ **Cholesterol** softens and smoothes out damage created in vascular walls.

➢ **Cholesterol** is a steroid precursor for hormones and cortisone.

➢ **Cholesterol** can be made by the body when more is needed.

➢ **Avoiding cholesterol** in the diet does not guarantee your cholesterol will be normal.

➢ **Cholesterol** medication damages the liver.

➢ **Cholesterol** can be made by cells for their own cell membranes.

End Notes

Nick, Gina L., Ph.D., N.D. *Clinical Purification*. Longevity Through Prevention, Inc., 2001.

8

Trans Fat Truth

Here is the chapter you have been waiting for, unless you skipped ahead. Naughty! Naughty! You need to go back if you did skip and get the full impact of what is to follow.

Scientists discovered that adding hydrogen at high temperatures to vegetable oil with the use of various catalysts would change the chemical property, bonds or hand holding, of fat molecules and atoms. Think back to the beginning of the explanation on fat. I discussed bonds, held hands, and the pliability and elasticity of the finished molecules of fatty acids. Saturated fat, one held hand or single bond, is generally hard and stiff at room temperature and can be heated without major change in configuration. Monounsaturated fat is one pair of held hands, or single double bond, and has more pliability and fluidity at room temperature. It is firm in cold temperatures, and can tolerate a moderate amount of heat. Polyunsaturated fats, like flax oil, with multiple pairs of held hands, are the most fragile and need to be kept cold where they will still retain their liquid form.

A few points to add to your understanding are that hydrogen and oxygen are also a part of the molecular structure of the fatty acid chains. Polyunsaturated fats are pliable and tend to bend on themselves or appear in a C or Cis position. When the heat and hydrogen are added to the vegetable oil at high temperatures, **there is a flip of one of the hands,** like twisting your wrist backwards, to add the hydrogen. **This results in a T configuration, or trans configuration, of the**

molecular shape. This also changes the consistency of the prior liquid oil to a firmer substance, margarine without cholesterol. **The new substance is now a saturated trans fat and all man-made trans fats are bad!!**

> **Every cell in your body has fat in it.**

Your body uses fats in cell membrane formation. Every cell in your body has fat in it. **The trans fat T confuses the system. Regardless of your training and who you are, trans fat is not health promoting.** The deal is, you cannot get away with fooling Mother Nature very long. The body will start to respond and react and over time breakdown. Trans fat, please

> **Trans fat, please recall, interferes with your body's making of PG1 and PG3, the pain relieving prostaglandins.**

recall, interferes with your body's production of PG1 and PG3, the pain relieving prostaglandins. You need more of those to balance the PG2, which is stimulated or enhanced by trans fat.

Producing parts for repair and function requires time just like making a luscious meal. The frame of time I have brought to your attention is the half life of trans fat. **The time to synthesize and process the man-made mutation is 51 days. That means in three months from the time you consume trans fat, you're still dealing with it.** Now, I also want you to be aware that the half life for Cis fat is 18 days. This means the essential fat takes eighteen days to be properly processed into cell membranes and have an effect on the body. I'm sure that you're not doing cart wheels over that tidbit of information either. The significance is when I make suggestions to my patients about health issues related to function dependent on fat, like hot flashes, ADHD, headaches, skin rashes, I tell them to be patient, an uncommon American virtue. **It will take a minimum of 18 days to see results.** Time and time again, three weeks into the protocol and BANG! the fat kicks in and they see the beginning of health restoration.

I normally as an aside, tell patients if they deviate from their diet by eating foods with trans fat, they should take a salmon capsule at night to counteract the drain on healthy tissue-supporting fat reserves. Salmon oil is a direct source of DHA and EPA (see Chapter 5). Now you should be seeing why people can consume a diet that causes or relieves pain. Got it?!

Trans fat is also found in limited amounts in nature. Your body generally, unless you overdose on that trans fat, will use it for energy and not cell membrane or tissue repair. People, especially younger people, consume more trans fat than Cis fat. It is no wonder why we have so many health ailments at younger and younger ages.

Let me throw one more little piece of information at you. I have been purposely using the term trans fat, trying to keep it simple by not using the word hydrogenated or partially hydrogenated fat. **Here is the bomb.** The process of changing or hydrogenating fat, if carried out to the full, will result in a product that is firm and hard and not necessarily suited for a wide spectrum of use. **Partial hydrogenation is when the process is stopped prematurely before complete hydrogenation occurs.** Food manufacturers prefer partially hydrogenated fat. Now, from all that I have observed over time, no one really knows what is created in the partial hydrogenation process. At least it won't be on the front page of a health magazine or journal. The travesty is, we have had an unsuspecting public, focused on "cholesterol free" for so long, that convincing them of the dangers of partial hydrogenation will be a monumental task. Then to add injury to insult, the facts are now being released that trans fat actually raises the level of LDL cholesterol and lowers HDL cholesterol. If that doesn't grab you in the throat, I don't know what will.

When reviewing the LDL/HDL issue with the ALA pathway and linoleic pathway, you find **that trans fat will raise the LDL level. This is the body's way of compensating. THE BODY IS TRYING TO SAVE ITSELF.** On the other hand, an inflamed and poorly functioning body needs to keep the HDL level low because its job is to take cholesterol out of vessels, but

With less sugar and reduced inflammation is a reduced need for LDL cholesterol.

it needs to be at the site of inflammation. I have used chromium in my practice for patients to reduce the craving for sugar which indirectly resets the HDL to naturally do its job because with less sugar and reduced inflammation is a reduced need for LDL cholesterol.

Summary

- ➤ **Cholesterol and saturated fat** are suspected to be the primary cause of heart disease.

- ➤ **Heated vegetable oil** has been the alternative to butter.

- ➤ **Heating vegetable oil** alters the consistency and property of the molecules confusing the body.

- ➤ **The body uses fat** to make cell membranes — man-made trans fat is not compatible for human function.

- ➤ **Trans fat** causes pain and inflammation and interferes with the formation of PG1 and PG3.

- ➤ **Partially hydrogenated fat** is a dirty bomb with negative residuals.

- ➤ **Sugar is the leading cause** of inflammation causing compensation with elevated LDL cholesterol used by the body to put the inflammation fire out.

- ➤ **Trans fat causes inflammation** by increasing PG2 and inhibiting PG1 and PG3.

9

Reading the Label Right

Did you ever get so upset that you wanted to shout? I believe the public needs to be screaming from the top of every building and mountain right now. The pharmaceutical and food manufacturers have been duping us for years. The desire to squeeze another buck out of the consumer, regardless of health consequences, perturbs me as a health care provider. The public has been eating low-fat and low-cholesterol for thirty years and yet obesity and cardiovascular disease are at all time highs. I have patients who, watching every item they eat, attempt to lower cholesterol based on recommendations of conventional medical thinking, yet they achieve little or no success. Why? Because the information they follow is wrong. Trying to avoid saturated fats in meat and dairy, people switched to eating vegetable based fat products containing trans fats, yet continue to be challenged with obesity and cardiovascular disease.

> **The pharmaceutical and food manufacturers have been duping us for years.**

Now, we have an opportunity to see the amount of trans fat in food on the labels of products. But are the labels telling the whole story? No, they only reveal a part of the picture. How much trans fat is safe? Should you eat an item that says no trans fat? Is there trans fat found in a package that boldly projects no trans fat? Here is an interesting point you should know. You

You should be eating less than one gram of man-made trans fat a day.

should be eating less than one gram of man-made trans fat a day. The food manufacturers have the permission to list 0 trans fat if the serving size of an item has less than 0.5 g of trans fat in it.

Now here is a big point: it was reported in the New England Journal of Medicine in 1997, that among 90,000 nurses studied, consuming 1.0 g or more of trans fat per day could increase your risk of heart or cardiovascular disease by 20 percent. Let's talk about this. Many lives should have been saved if this was a daily public service announcement like the "Just Say No" campaign against drugs, smoking or alcohol. Now you can see why I am concerned about your health.

Remember, I see real patients every day who are living with surgical scars zigzagging across their chests, abdomens, and trunks from heart and gall bladder operations and who ate what they were told was safe. You can now purchase a bag of snack food that literally has only one half gram or less of trans fat per serving! The key word is per serving — eat the whole addictive bag of "junk food" and you will consume five or six grams of trans fat. You think you are eating no trans fat and are safe.

Over time, because of the long half life which translates to a long shelf life of trans fat, you have essential fatty acid physiology that has broken down, as symptoms of pain, headaches, skin rashes, asthma, depression, and fibromyalgia appear. You retrace what you have been eating, and think, hey, I'm doing really good. It must be something I inherited. Wrong! **You have been feeding your system a toxin that interferes with all membrane function.**

Probably the most confusion is going to be the labels that say no trans fat. They legitimately may have no trans fat, but have any number of experimental fats in the ingredients you have not heard of yet. A worse case scenario will be the new, man-made, untested substitute fats. Even though they are not a trans fat, they still have the potential to interfere with your body's ability to properly utilize essential fatty acids. I honestly do not think there will ever be a totally 100 percent safe, effective man-made substitute fat. I can confidently say that because I treat real people and not lab animals. Real people can food journal, and I can correlate symptoms and bodily dysfunction with patterns of foods consumed. Patients who eat out, and at least 20 percent of Americans eat out daily, and more than 30 percent of our youth eat at fast food restaurants every day, are consuming **heated fats, and heated fat is a part of the experience.** Patients who visit my office with poor health and severe body signals from relentless migraines to cancer, **always** have a history of eating items that interfere with fat metabolism.

Man-made, or natural fats which are chemically or physically altered, interfere with the body's function at the cellular level. You will — I promise — have some type of dysfunction if you focus on foods that have heated fats as a part of the ingredients. Stealthily hidden fats, or obvious ones, can disrupt your ability to function and medication alleviates symptoms only temporarily.

So what do you need to do? Become a student of label reading. The following common questions on the FDA's labeling of trans fatty acids will assist your ability to decipher foods that are packaged. Restaurants are not required to follow the trans fat labeling rule. Trans fat, regardless of the source, is not safe. It has been suggested that one percent or less of your daily fat can be trans fat. I would strongly encourage you to focus on consuming natural, whole foods without added man-made oils versus convenience packaged items. Buyer beware!

Nutrition Facts		
Serving Size 28/About 15 chips		
Servings Per Container 11		

Amount Per Serving	
Calories 150 Calories from Fat 90	
	% Daily Value*
Total Fat 10g	15%
Saturated Fat 3g	15%
Trans Fat 0g	
Cholesterol 0mg	0%
Sodium 200mg	3%
Total Carbohydrate 15g	5%
Dietary Fiber 1g	4%
Sugars 2g	
Protein 2g	

Vitamin A 0%	•	Vitamin C 10%
Calcium 0 %	•	Iron 0%
Vitamin E 6%	•	Thiamin 4%
Niacin 6%	•	Vitamin B6 4%
Phosphorus 4%	•	Zinc 2%

		Calories	2,000	2,500
Total Fat	Less than	65g	80g
Sat Fat	Less than	20g	25g
Cholesterol	Less than	300mg	300mg
Sodium	Less than	2,400mg	2,400mg
Total Carbohydrate		300g	375g
Dietary Fiber		25g	30g

Ingredients: Partially Hydrogenated (Soybean and Canola Oils)

According to the FDA, the amount of trans fat in a serving will be listed below the saturated fat listing on a food label. What the FDA will not do is give trans fat a %Daily Value (%DV) as it does on all other vitamins and minerals contained in a product. Because of the relationship between trans fat and heart disease, no daily amount will be listed. However, saturated fats will still be given a daily amount since the amount you can eat safely has been established as between 5-20 percent.

The question arises: is it possible for a food product to list the amount of trans fat as 0g on the Nutrition Facts panel even if the ingredient list contains partially hydrogenated vegetable oil? That answer is yes since only an amount of 0.5 grams or more is required to be listed. So relatively speaking you could be consuming 5 grams of trans fat every day if you eat 10 products that contain trans fat even though it is less than 0.5 grams per serving. The moral of this story is read the ingredients list and not just the Nutrition Facts label!

The FDA has listed what they refer to as highlights to the trans fat rule. The first is that manufacturers of convenient foods and some dietary supplements need to list trans fat on a separate line immediately under saturated fat on the nutrition label. Next, the FDA has established the definition for trans fat to be "all unsaturated fatty acids that contain one or more isolated double bond in a trans configuration." And lastly, dietary supplement manufacturers must also list trans fat on the Supplement Facts panel when their products contain reportable amounts, 0.5 grams or more, of trans fat such as in energy and nutrition bars. What about dietary supplements? Do they also contain trans fat? The answer is yes, some dietary supplements do contain ingredients that include partially hydrogenated vegetable oil or trans fat as well as saturated fat and cholesterol. As a result of the FDA's new label requirement, if a dietary supplement contains a reportable amount of trans fat, which is 0.5 grams or more, dietary supplement manufacturers must list the amounts on the Supplement Facts panel. Examples of dietary supplements that may contain saturated fat, trans fat, and cholesterol include energy and nutrition bars.

Concerning the heart disease and trans fat connection, the FDA relied on scientific reports, expert panels, and studies from the Institute of Medicine/National Academies of Science and the National Cholesterol Education Program as well as the DHHS and the USDA which conclude that consumption of trans fatty acids contribute to increased LDL levels thus increasing coronary heart disease. They strongly encourage that trans fat consumption be as low as possible and to use liquid vegetable oil and soft margarine instead of butter, stick margarine, and shortening. It is my opinion that you should do everything possible to keep trans fat consumption to the least amount possible. The challenge appears when you eat out at a restaurant. The fast food and local diners do not have to post the amount of trans fat. Remember, American teens eat out almost daily and trans fat is lurking in nearly every item they choose.

Americans teens eat out almost daily and trans fat is lurking in nearly every item they choose.

This article appeared on August 18, 2005 at
www.newsday.com/news/health/ny-hsfries0818,0,652990.story
©2005, Newsday, Inc.
By staff writer Roni Rabin

Study finds link between fries and breast cancer

A study examining the role childhood diet plays in breast cancer has found an association between eating French fries regularly during the preschool years and developing breast cancer as an adult.

Each weekly serving of French fries girls consumed between ages 3 and 5 increased their risk of developing breast cancer as adults by 27 percent, according to researchers at Brigham and Women's Hospital and the Harvard School of Public Health.

The association was not found with potatoes prepared in other ways.

The finding is the first of its kind and must be confirmed by other studies, said lead author Karin Michels, an associate professor at Harvard Medical School and clinical epidemiologist at Brigham and Women's Hospital in Boston.

"This is something nobody's really looked at before. It's really new," she said, adding, "It could be due to chance."

The finding of a correlation between French fries and breast cancer does not necessarily point to a cause-and-effect relationship between the two, however.

Michels speculated the French fries may be implicated in breast cancer because they are prepared in fats that are high in harmful trans-fatty acids and saturated fat.

The dietary survey examined the childhood eating habits of participants in the Harvard Nurses' Health Study. To obtain information about what adult women had eaten as preschoolers, the researchers asked the mothers of participants in the nurses' study to fill out questionnaires asking how often their daughters had eaten 30 different food items.

The researchers analyzed data gathered in 1993 from 582 participants with breast cancer and 1,569 women without breast cancer. The participants were born between 1921 and 1965, so their mothers were being asked to recall information from decades earlier.

Michels noted these recollections may have been unreliable, especially when made by mothers who already knew their daughters had breast cancer.

Consumption of whole milk was associated with a slightly decreased risk of breast cancer, though most of the milk consumed during those decades was whole milk, Michels said.

"Only one food so distinctly stood out as being associated with breast cancer risk," Michels said, and that was the French fries.

She said dietary influences may be more significant during early life than during adulthood, because the breast of a girl or infant is more susceptible to environmental influences than the breast of a mature woman.

Dr. Larry Norton, deputy physician in chief of the breast cancer program at Memorial Sloan-Kettering Cancer Center in New York, warned against over-interpreting the results.

"I wouldn't go out and change Americans' dietary habits on the basis of this, but it's certainly worth pursuing the hypothesis with additional research," he said.

Michels said her study doesn't prove that giving up French fries will protect against breast cancer.

But with child obesity rates rising, she said, "There are numerous reasons to avoid French fries."

10

Winning the Pain Game

It is estimated that 50 to 80 percent of our population suffers with pain on a daily basis creating a multi-billion dollar pharmaceutical industry. There are many reasons for pain. Did you know that what you eat will control pain levels in your body? The consumption of trans fat is one of several factors that promotes pain by increasing the production of a fat tissue hormone discussed earlier (see Chapter 4) called prostaglandin 2 (PG2), or by inhibiting the body's ability to make pain relieving prostaglandin 1 (PG1), and prostaglandin 3 (PG3). Pain is an integral part of normal bodily function. When a body part is damaged by injury from a fall, motor vehicle accident, sports injury, etc., chemicals are released to **stimulate the healing process.** Your body is specifically designed to repair itself. We are a self-healing organism and pain is part of the process. You naturally will tend to favor an injured area as the body goes about its business of damage control. There is a specific set of natural steps that occur. Pain can also occur because of postural breakdown during the aging process. Aging tissues are compressed, stretched, squeezed and moved, creating a bombardment to the supporting structures. This results in a chemical release response causing repair from an injury to be slower and more painful. Chronic pain syndromes are a common unresolved dilemma.

> **Did you know that what you eat will control pain levels in your body?**

> **Pain is an integral part of normal bodily function.**

The million dollar question for chronic pain sufferers is: what causes the pain? This is the most obvious question to answer, but from my point, it is the one that has not been addressed because of the general public's ignorance and the greed of those in the conventional pain relieving market. The accepted mindset is that it is easier to take a pill to relieve pain than it is to make lifestyle changes to alleviate the pain altogether.

Pain is real. I have seen thousands of patients who have had pain for years find relief in a short time period without adding a new medication. Pain at the cellular level is caused by uncontrolled chemical responses precipitated by eating foods that inhibit PG1 and/or PG3 production so they cannot be a part of the pain relieving equation. Another factor in the pain relieving equation is in eating too much of the foods that create PG1 (safflower and sunflower oils, snack and convenience foods). When these are in overabundance in the body, PG2 is created, adding pain instead of relieving it (see Chart 2 on page 29). This information is not currently commonly known or understood, or perhaps, because it seems so simple, it is just ignored. After all, many still think margarine is good.

What foods cause pain? Foods that stop PG1 and PG3. The number one and two foods are trans fat and sugar which are in nearly all prepackaged snack food products. Trans fat prolongs pain because of its 51 day half-life. Your body is concentrating on trying to metabolize the trans fat that inhibits the pain-relieving prostaglandins. Your body goes out of balance. You need to consume a 1:1 ratio of Omega-6 fats which produce PG1 and Omega-3 fats which produce PG3. A ratio of 4:1 is a logical goal to begin relieving some of the pain. You at least won't have relentless pain with a 4:1 ratio. Here is the new millennium challenge: ask your physician about fat and pain relief. Don't be surprised if you get the deer-in-the-headlights stare. Most health care providers do not know that fat is part of the pain-relief equation.

When the ratio is 1:1 to 4:1, there is an even distribution of pain relief and pain causing chemicals. A common occurrence in America with our addiction to snack foods is more like 20:1. Yes, the public eats twenty times the amount of foods that

The public eats twenty times the amount of foods that cause pain versus relieve pain.

cause pain versus relieve pain. And that is why the pain relief industry is so huge! That huge disparity also contributes to blood vessel inflammation with high LDL cholesterol as well as other behavioral, emotional, and memory dysfunctions (see Chapter 11).

Now, take a look at the following chart and see the foods that contribute to the various prostaglandins.

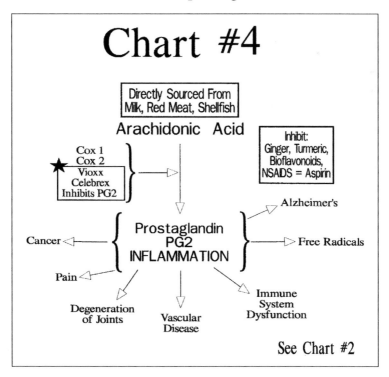

Take a look at snack food and energy bar labels. You can easily see why what we are eating is causing our pain. Most of our snack foods contain dairy, sugar and trans fat, and many of us over eat meat which adds to the pain. Excessive PG2 can create an environment increasing not only pain and vascular disease, but also cancer, decay, immune system dysfunctions, free radicals (think oxidation damage like rusting), and Alzheimer's (see Chart #4). Pain relievers work by interfering with the production of PG2. When the PG2 pathway is altered, there is a cascade effect altering the ratio of PG1 and PG3.

Before I made Dr. DeMaria's recommended lifestyle changes, I was suffering with TMJ pain, pain in my arms, occasional back pain, digestive problems, and seasonal depression that was encouraged by pain. Following Dr.'s advice I began to exercise, stopped drinking milk and coffee, started eating more organic foods when possible and began taking recommended vitamins, flax oil and salmon oil. It has been difficult to change my schedule to allow time for exercise. I no longer take Vioxx and Wellbutrin. I am now much better able to handle the "winter blues" without pain. I feel pretty much pain free. I feel much better about not taking medications and hope to limit my use of prescription medications.

~Karen Netherland

Taking medication to stop pain without thinking about what is causing the pain is similar to taking pharmaceuticals to lower

LDL cholesterol without attempting to correct the cause. A side note: the pharmaceutical companies, in all due respect, encourage dietary changes in the advertising and marketing campaigns. The public avoids cholesterol foods like cheese, ice cream and red meat which is a step in the right direction. The real cause of high cholesterol and pain is, however, sugar, vitamin and mineral deficiencies, and trans fat, and these issues are not being presented.

Prostaglandin #1 Primarily sourced from Omega 6 fats	Prostaglandin #2 Primarily sourced from Omega 6 fats and directly from the following:	Prostaglandin #3 Primarily sourced from Omega 6 fats
☑ Primrose Oil ☑ Black Currant Oil ☑ Borage Oil ☑ Safflower Oil ☑ Sunflower Oil	☑ Dairy ☑ Red Meat ☑ Mollusks ☑ Shellfish	☑ Flax Oil ☑ Greens ☑ Algae ☑ Selected nuts ☑ Fish - directly sourced from fish

Now, you know that trans fat can precipitate pain and eating too many trans fat alternative fats like safflower and sunflower can also cause pain because they are part of the Omega-6 family. Remember the ratio is the key. Omega-6 fats are not bad for you, but the amount must be balanced with Omega-3 fats for our bodies to function properly. Margarine is almost purely an Omega-6 fatty acid, yet it is a trans fat. It should not be anywhere near your diet!

Margarine is almost purely an Omega-6 fatty acid and it is a trans fat. It should not be anywhere near your diet!

You have now been empowered to know what causes pain. So what do you do? You first of all avoid pain promoting sugar, dairy, trans fats, and sweet fruits like bananas, raisins, grapes, pineapple and dried fruits. Introduce Omega-3 foods like mixed green salads, green beans, walnuts, flax oil, flax seeds and flax powder into your diet. Also consume vitamin B rich foods and minerals, including zinc, magnesium and calcium. Alfalfa is a good source of all these minerals. Work on replacing dairy with rice, almond and oat milk products. In my office, we do not encourage soy products. Soy can deplete zinc and encourage aluminum to remain in the body, neither of which promotes optimal health. Choose to eat a variety of fresh, raw organic vegetables and the fruits such as pears, plums and apples. Grains have a ratio of 20:1 or greater and grain-fed animals have ratios above 4:1. In the pain equation, these should be referred to as pro-inflammatory foods.

For those of you taking a COX drug, how does this affect you? COX is an acronym for cyclo-oxygenase. Much has been discussed about COX-1 and COX-2. It has also been proposed there is a COX-3. The difference between the first two is straight forward. COX-1 is an enzyme involved in bodily functions like stomach protection and kidney function. In contrast COX-2 is not involved at all in tissue function or balance; instead it is induced or active after tissue injury.

There is confusion revolving around COX-2 being an inflammatory enzyme. It is not. COX-2 is an enzyme that is induced by tissue injury. The response is dependent on the nature of the fatty acids present in the cell membranes. This is huge, huge, HUGE. The response is determined by what you are eating!! If COX-2 acts with arachidonic acid, the outcome will be the synthesis of PG2 which produces pain, reduces blood flow, and causes blood platelets to stick. If the fat to make PG1 or DGLA is present, there is a non-inflammatory response. If the fat to make PG3 or EPA is present, there is a non-inflammatory response. Pharmacology articles and pathology texts do not make this distinction which is why the public is led to believe that COX-2 enzymes are inherently inflammatory*. The bad effects of the COX inhibiting medication is a travesty. I have personally witnessed and talked with patients who have had spinal cord strokes directly related to this type of pain reliever. Tens of thousands of people have been harmed.

We literally eat ourselves into a state of inflammation and pain and then have to take medications as a counteractive measure. The excessive inflammation created by the overabundance of Omega-6 fatty acids is also thought to be the

> **The excessive inflammation created by the overabundance of Omega-6 fatty acids is also thought to be the main reason for the development of cancer, heart disease, stroke, and other inflammatory conditions.**

main reason for the development of cancer, heart disease, stroke, and other inflammatory conditions. The headlines in major newspapers consistently report the new information being released on the dangers of cox medications, plus aspirin and other non-steroidal anti-inflammatory drugs. A word of caution — think twice before you put a pain reliever in your body.

End Notes

*CSPI. "Researchers Failed to Gauge COX-2 Heart-Attack Risks, Despite Early Warnings." February 16, 2005. {online}. Available: http://www.cspinet.org. February 16, 2005.

Trans Fat a Cause of OBESITY?

According to the American Obesity Association, 127 million adults in the United States are overweight, while 60 million are obese and 9 million are severely obese. Much to do with the dangerous belly fat common in overweight and obese Americans.

A new Wake Forest University study shows that trans fats also largely contribute to dangerous belly fat. The six-year study tracked the health changes of 51 male vervet monkeys that were split into two groups and fed identical diets, but with one difference: One group got 8 percent of its calories from trans fats, while the other group received those calories from healthy monounsaturated fats, such as olive oil.

By the end of the study, the monkeys fed the trans fats had increased their body weight by 7.2 percent versus the other group, which only experienced a 1.8 percent increase. However, the most telling difference between the two groups was easy to see: The trans fat monkeys had grown large bellies, while the other group had not. Researchers said the weight gain was surprising, since neither group had been fed enough calories to gain weight — especially not the 30 percent increase in abdominal fat that the trans fat group experienced.

In addition, the researchers found that the trans fats not only caused excess visceral fat; they actually caused fat from other parts of the body to be redistributed to the belly. Researchers concluded that, calorie for calorie, consuming trans fats leads to greater weight gain, especially in the belly area.

Though sporting a large belly is generally considered a social taboo in the United States, it's also one of the most dangerous manifestations of obesity. Research in the last few years has revealed that wide girths often indicate large quantities of visceral fat, which is the deeply hidden fat surrounding the organs in the abdominal region. Visceral fat has been linked with high insulin levels, high cholesterol, high triglycerides, and high blood pressure, as well as a host of other ailments.

Even for those who are just a few pounds overweight and lack the telltale belly often associated with high visceral fat levels, the amount of hidden fat can be surprisingly high. For example, seniors should be especially careful to keep a slim abdomen, since even normal-weight seniors with larger amounts of hidden visceral fat run an increased risk of developing type 2 diabetes.

Six years of fast-food fats supersizes monkeys, *New Scientist* Issue 2556 17 June 2006, page 21

11

ADHD to Alzheimer's: The Trans Fat Connection

The fact that your body needs quality fat to function should not be a surprise to you at this point, unless of course you scanned the table of contents and came to this chapter first!

I did a pilot study several years ago to test a hypothesis I developed concerning behavior dysfunction including ADHD, ADD, hyperactivity, and Oppositional Defiant Disorder (ODD). The thought came to me after looking at a map that was in *USA Today* revealing the pounds of snack food consumed in various geographic centers in the US. The Midwest and North Central part of America consumed the most, nearly twenty-four pounds per person each year. I am sure the pounds of snacks are well over thirty pounds each by now. I also was aware through the Drug Enforcement Agency, DEA, that Ritalin at one point was being used by over eight percent of school children in Northern Michigan. Martha's Vineyard was a close second. With those statistics correlating with the volume of snacks consumed being the highest in those areas, I knew there was a connection.

Ritalin is a schedule II drug, which means it has to be accounted for and requires an assessment to be prescribed.

Ritalin is a schedule II drug, which means it has to be accounted for and requires an assessment to be prescribed. It has similar characteristics as cocaine. **There was one point where school nurses or principal's offices had more Ritalin on hand than did the local pharmacies!** The Southern areas in the US including Florida and California did not use the same magnitude of Ritalin according to the DEA, nor did they consume the amount of snack foods as other areas in the US did.

The metabolism of fat for the brain was and is being altered by something. Decision makers did not and have not correlated trans fat with the production of docosahexaenoic acid (DHA) by the ALA pathway (see Chapter 4). Trans fat only recently has been recognized as a part of the heart disease equation that stimulated trans fat labeling. DHA is needed for brain function. Eicosapentaenoic acid, EPA, is the long chain fat needed for heart health. It is also affected in a negative way by trans fat. **Information available suggests that eating only one gram of trans fat per day can increase your potential to create the environment for cardiovascular challenges by 20 percent.** The frightening news is that labeling of serving sizes of one-half gram or less can be considered as having no trans fat. Something is not right with this equation (see page 68).

The pilot program for ADHD that I developed and completed was for 102 days and is described in detail in Chapter 18 of *Dr. Bob's Guide to Stop ADHD in 18 Days*. It demonstrated that, yes, the correct diet modifications can improve and relieve symptoms of ADHD in 18 days. The eighteen days is the half life of Cis fat metabolism (see page 62). I met regularly with a group of children and adults for four months. I required the participants to eliminate dairy and trans fat from their diets. They consumed sugar alternatives (see page 106). The group took whole food B vitamins, minerals, flax oil, and salmon oil. They only took the salmon oil which is a direct source of DHA for 18 days. We had a huge celebration only three weeks into the program. Some of the surprising results included symptoms of thunderstorm static noises that went away, behavior being quieted, and an overall sense of calmness occurring. Why?

Your body needs a quality source of food to thrive. It can survive for a season on processed devitalized ingredients, but over time, the system breaks down. Children's brains need fat to grow and work optimally. Boys require three times the amount of fat compared to their female counterparts. That is a reason why you will see more young men having behavior issues than girls. Teenage young men also consume more soda than young women do. Soda has sugar; sugar interferes with DHA production. Finally, **today one third of all American youths and children from 4-19 are estimated to eat at fast food restaurants.** They will order food fried in fat, eat grains with a high ratio of Omega-6 to Omega-3 or at least above the optimal 4:1 ratio (see page 74), and/or have a milk shake or ice cream novelty item.

In his book *Fast Food Nation*, Eric Schlosser states that your French fries go through a more thorough examination than you do when you get a physical. They are analyzed, altered, and made perfect for consumption and then they are fried in hydrogenated oil. These patterns create a scenario for disaster. With the amount of fast food America eats — it is estimated at three hamburgers and four orders of fries weekly — we are packing our bodies with synthetics and hydrogenated oils resulting in unhealthy bodies and hyperactive children. What is even more interesting is the nearly 5 million plus ADHD youths will become ADHD adults. It is estimated over 60 percent of youths diagnosed with ADHD translates to an accumulated 8 million adults over time. The process does not stop. The adults with ADHD may not recognize they still have the condition or are in denial and become depressed.

Eighteen percent of Americans, at least 50 million, take anti-depressants. The physiology from my experience is the same. The improper metabolism of fat and slowing or stopping DHA creates short circuits in the brain and nerves leading to ADHD and depression.

Why does this happen? Your body sends messages on a layer of fat called the myelin sheath. Quality nutrients are required, not suggested, for this to occur in a timely, uninterrupted manner. Your body takes the food you eat and attempts through steps to make items necessary for all functions. **Trans fat interferes with your body's ability to make the fat needed for proper brain and emotional activity.**

Convenience food is heavy on trans fat and Omega-6 fat (safflower and sunflower oils).

We live in a fast-paced society. Convenience food is heavy on trans fat and Omega-6 fat (safflower and sunflower oils). These do not promote DHA fat (see Chart #3, page 42). The predominately popular low fat diet has permeated our culture for thirty years. Low fat meant high trans fat (vegetable oil with no cholesterol) and high carbohydrates (loaded with sugar). **This formula has been the death sentence for two generations.** Both ingredients, the trans fat and sugar, have slipped under the radar, stopping our bodies from working efficiently and creating a staircase crescendo of ADHD, depression, pain syndromes and finally, the last curtain call — Alzheimer's. Just the mention of the term Alzheimer's can stop the best. Take a look at some Alzheimer's statistics:

➢ Women with Alzheimer's tend to live longer than men (*USA Today*, 2004).

➢ The severity of Alzheimer's is the most important predictor of length of survival.

➢ When tested, people with poor initial memory tests had a high risk of dying quickly; perhaps the disease was advanced at the time of the diagnosis.

> It is estimated 16 million Americans will develop Alzheimer's by 2050.

The patterns that develop in youth continue on into adulthood. The seniors today lived through the low fat high carbohydrate mania. Omega-3 fat from the ALA pathway is not as effective today because of trans fat and critically low mineral and vitamin levels. Seniors do not always eat quality food. It is easier to heat up a dinner for one than make something from scratch. A recent study reported that Omega-3 fats help the nerve charges on seniors. The seniors studied with higher Omega-3 food had reduced symptoms of Alzheimer's versus those who consumed the standard American diet (*USA Today*, 2003).

A recent study reported that Omega-3 fats help the nerve charges on seniors.

Are you getting it? The physiology is the same. It has been suggested that eating fish, a direct source of Omega-3 fats, can help prevent or stop Alzheimer's. Here is my suggestion; are you ready for this pearl of wisdom? Your goal is to focus on creating DHA for brain function and EPA for heart function by observing and respecting the body's ability to make DHA and EPA from the food you eat and not from fish oil exclusively. You can eat fish if you want and take salmon capsules, one every two or three days, but the best to do is this — eat a mixed green salad with chicken or turkey protein daily. Protein is needed to make neurotransmitters. Use flax oil as a part of the dressing. Avoid dairy and sugar. Eat walnuts and green beans. Alfalfa sprouts are a good mineral source. Olive oil is great for sautéing food. Fresh organic eggs are the best. Vary your breads using spelt, rye, oat and sprouted grain which are excellent. Be sensitive to the amount of Omega-6 fats you consume. Vary your grains. Do not eat wheat exclusively. Whole food B vitamins, B6, minerals and flax oil are essential. Concentrate on fresh, raw, organic or steamed vegetables; do not boil them to death. Animal protein is okay, but limit red meat, not avoid it. Avoid and eliminate pork. Soy has an affinity for aluminum and should be limited to eight ounces or less daily. Our society eats the same amount of fish today as we did in the 1970s. The public doesn't need to increase their intake of fish. **You need to avoid trans fat with its long half life.** Do not lose sleep over someone telling you that Alzheimer's is inherited. Focus on changing the diet pattern you are following if it is the same as your loved one who has Alzheimer's.

My parents have issues with emotional distress like some of you. My dad is addicted to doughnuts, sugar and ice cream. My mom can't miss sugar at a meal. They are in denial. You may be in denial. This is not a game. My mom doesn't even remember what she ate for breakfast. You do not need to be like your parents. My wife and I follow the plan I previously detailed. It works! I have been involved with natural, drugless care for over 30 years and have helped prevent many, many thousands of patients from having emotional meltdowns. By the way, you can deviate from the plan, just don't let the exception become the rule.

Regardless of what you may read in the media, your body, when given the right ingredients, has the innate ability to make what it needs to function optimally, genetically. We have not changed as a species, as some suggest. Most have been feeding their bodies wrongly. The established mindset still thinks the world is flat. Test me on this. No trans fat, no sugar, limited to no dairy for 102 days and see how you feel. You'll live to remember it forever.

Summary

> **Snack and convenience foods** made with trans fat interfere with the formation of DHA.

> **Ritalin** is a schedule II drug.

- **Salmon oil** is a direct source of DHA.

- **Young males** require 3 times the fat as young women do.

- **ADHD children** become ADHD adults more than 50 percent of the time.

- **Eighteen percent of the American public** takes anti-depressants.

- **Omega-6 fats** do not promote DHA for brain health.

- **Focus on eating mixed greens** for lunch.

- **We consume the same amount** of marine life as we did in the 1970s.

- **Avoid trans fat** with its long shelf life.

- **The same physiology leading to ADHD** translates to depression and finally Alzheimer's.

$\sim$

End Notes

Fackelman, Kathleen. "Alzheimer's Can Cut Life Expectancy in Half." *USA Today*. April 4, 2004.

Fackelman, Kathleen. "Fish Diet May Fight Alzheimer's." *USA Today*. July 22, 2003.

12

Trans Fat: The Saboteur to Your Health

The all important essential fatty acids and their complete metabolism to other critical components are necessary for life. You have discovered that common but poorly understood and treated conditions from ADHD to Alzheimer's are precipitated by improper fat formation. Trans fat interferes with health at the cell membrane level. The membrane is permeable like a sieve or screen on a door. Fluids can easily cross back and forth with nutrients and wastes. Trans fat formation literally hardens the cell membrane. Your chronic health conditions can be directly linked to the foods you choose or decide not to eat that interfere with this transmission.

Common but poorly understood and treated conditions from ADHD to Alzheimer's are precipitated by improper fat formation.

Trans fat has penetrated our society so deeply that nearly every item in a package has trans fat or partially hydrogenated fat as a primary ingredient. Trans fat has a long shelf life; remember the half life of trans fat is 51 days. Fat from animal sources becomes rancid quickly and needs to be refrigerated.

Trans fat has penetrated our society so deeply that nearly every item in a package has trans fat or partially hydrogenated fat as a primary ingredient.

Trans fat enhances pastries so they are flaky. My grandma's homemade donuts were always cooked in lard and they tasted best when they were freshly cooked. After that, they were as hard as a rock.

The real issue of your health and trans fat is the fact that the complete mechanism of the essential fats is disrupted with a cascade effect. What is important for you to grasp is first, you need to eat essential fats. Your body cannot make them. Essential fats are required for life. Second, items you eat like trans fat, sugar, dairy, aspirin, insulin stimulators, and steroids detour your body from maximizing their potential.

Essential fats are required for life.

This is about promoting life. I see patients every day who have severe long-term health maladies and who have been improperly evaluated. The conventional mindset always looks for an outside-in answer for an inside-out problem. I want to laugh at times when new patients recite the litany of the best doctors they have been to and the famous clinics and universities that look for answers in all the wrong places.

Today, powerful medications to numb and deaden the pain receptors are common. The ruthless side effects paralyze normal daily activity. Recently one young man presented my office with a two year history of "vice gripping" headaches that totally stopped his life. He listed his six medications and mentioned the famous institutions that he had visited without success. The medication they put him on was addictive and interfered with his work. They were planning on more medication. I took one look at him and immediately sized up the situation. He had "Uncle Fester" eyes, from the Adams Family. He acknowledged my observation. I learned he had two passions — junk food and dairy. Dairy, from my experience, always causes dark circles under the eyes. The trans fats, together with the dairy, interrupted his production of prostaglandin 3 (PG3) that relieves pain and inflammation. Headaches can be precipitated by any food made with trans fat and junk food can be addictive. He was ignorant of this cause and effect.

Essential fats cannot be made by the body. They are required for healthy cells and are necessary for production of hormones, proteins, prostaglandins and neurotransmitters. These four items, when out of synchronicity, are the cause of nearly every health issue, either directly or indirectly, by interfering with function. Even what seems so insignificant at the cell level can cause chronic severe headaches that will not go away unless you change the cause. Pain relievers do not treat causes.

Possible conditions as a result of the breakdown of essential fat metabolism due to consuming trans fats:

> Gritty or dry eyes

> Glandular problems including:

  Adrenal insufficiency

  Miscarriages

  Infertility

  PMS

  Growth impairment

> Hair problems:

  Alopecia or patchy hair loss

  Brittle hair

  Unmanageable hair

  Split ends

> Healing issues:

  Bleeding gums

  Delayed wound healing

  Intolerance or slow recovery from exercise

  Nosebleeds

> Heart issues:

  Hardening of the arteries

  Heart disease

> Intestinal issues:

  Chronic diarrhea

  Chrohn's disease

  Irritable bowel syndrome

- Mental issues:
  - Alzheimer's
  - Anxiety/depression
  - ADHD
  - Autism
  - Dementia
  - Headaches
  - Irritability and/or nervousness
  - Memory loss
  - Parkinson's disease
  - Retardation
  - Seizures
  - Senility
  - Violent behavior
- Metabolic problems:
  - Loss of appetite
  - Obesity
  - Unexplained weight loss
  - Brittle nails
- Asthma
- Emphysema
- Skin problems:
  - Acne
  - Dermatitis
  - Dry, flaky skin
  - Dry or oily skin
  - Dryness or cracks behind ears
  - Dry patches of skin on face or nose
  - Easy bruising
  - Eczema
  - Enlarged facial pores
  - Constantly chapped lips
  - Psoriasis
  - Seborrhea
- Dry mouth or throat especially when speaking
- Tingling in the arms and legs
- Urinary problems including bladder infections and chronic kidney disease
- Alcoholism
- Arthritis
- Cancer
- Diabetes
- Lupus
- Sjoren's syndrome

To remedy these symptoms, I encourage my patients to take 1 tablespoon of flax oil per 100 pounds of weight on a daily basis. I also encourage them to eliminate all trans fats from their diets. My patients who follow this simple plan see their symptoms lessen or disappear because fats are properly metabolized, their body fat decreases, and their organs begin to function healthfully.

Before making Dr. DeMaria's recommended lifestyle changes my skin would not heal, I had knee pain when I walked or ran, and I had numbness in both hands. I also had visual disturbances and headaches that occurred often. I had also invested in many topicals from dermatologists that didn't help and I also took oral antibiotics. It has been difficult, but I have eliminated most sugar from my diet and now take a zinc supplement, flax oil and vitamins. The information provided by Dr. Bob has improved my life. My health has improved and has given me hope for further improvements. I have given my testimony to many friends and family and hope that they find their way here!

Laura Lackas

Allergies are a common problem. The precipitating factor for many health issues including allergies is inflammation. Trans fat interferes with pain relieving PG3. Intestinal lining can become inflamed with tiny holes. Incompletely digested, or poorly digested food particles especially protein, commonly the difficult to digest casein, dairy protein in milk, slips through the holes. The body sees the protein as a foreign invader. A reaction occurs and histamines are released to control and dilute the attack. You have phlegm, post nasal drip, chronic cough, sneezing, and on and on. You seek help; an anti-histamine is prescribed. You feel fine for a season — then the bad effects from medication start, including dry mouth, eyes and nose. Drowsiness occurs and you don't feel quite 100 percent. Then you stop the meds and the initial symptoms return and you are beside yourself, not knowing what to do. Common scenario? You bet! I see it every day and have for years. The little holes in the intestine create an environment for a host of conditions. **Poor digestion means you are not**

absorbing what your body needs in order to thrive. You get tired; your hair falls out and you cry easily without reason. You feel depressed, sluggish and in pain. Is an anti-depressant your answer? No.

You would do best to follow my advice. Avoid items that interfere with the formation of PG3, EPA and DHA. Trans fat by far is the single biggest threat to your health. Current **Trans fat by far is the single biggest threat to your health.** convenience food is heavily weighted with addictive taste enhancers that are excitotoxins to the brain. This, with trans fat, sugar, and food colors, inhibits optimal health.

One last thought. Trans fat over time will be replaced by some other man-made fat. Be watchful. Trans fat was heavily endorsed for over 30 years before it was accepted to be the problem. It was created to be the savior and is determined to be the silent killer. Heating oils always changes the composition. Do not focus on alternatives and avoid fried items. There are other possibilities. Focus on fresh organic vegetables — raw or steamed, organic meat, pure water and whole-grain, sprouted grain bread. Eggs are your friend. Oatmeal with almonds is a great way to start the day. You might want to change the breakfast cereal and milk habit. Dairy can be your problem, interrupting PG3 production, something unknown by most people. Avoiding trans fats is part of a hormone-healthy diet.

Summary

➤ Trans fat sabotages the production of DHA, EPA, and PG3.

➤ The half life of trans fat is 51 days.

➤ Trans fat stimulates the production of painful PG2.

Adverse Effects of Trans Fats

1. Damage to the functions of cell membranes, when trans fats become part of membrane structure. Because cells are responsible for transporting nutrients, hormones and waste products, cells become "stupid" when membranes have absorbed trans fats.

2. Negatively affects fat-based steroid hormone balance and levels.

3. Increases insulin levels in the blood and contributes to insulin resistance.

4. Decreases the response of the red blood cells to insulin and contributes even more to insulin resistance.

5. Escalates the adverse effects of essential fatty acid EFA deficiency.

6. Blocks the conversion of Omega-6 and Omega-3 EFAs into their elongated fatty acids and eicosanoids (cellular hormones).

7. Increases total cholesterol

8. Decreases HDLs and increases LDLs in a dose-dependent manner meaning the more trans fat you eat, the more it disrupts your cholesterol balance.

9. Raises the atherosclerosis forming repair protein, whereas saturated fats lower this repair protein. This means that trans fats irritate the inner artery walls and saturated fats protect them which is just the opposite of industry propaganda.

10. Lowers the volume of cream and the quality of breast milk.

11. Correlates with low infant birth weight.

12. Decreases visual acuity in infants in a dose-dependent manner when they are fed breast milk containing trans fat.

13. Precipitates childhood asthma.

14. Weakens immunity.

15. Causes adverse alterations in enzymes that metabolize carcinogens.

16. Causes enlargement of adipose cell size, cell number, lipid class, and fatty acid composition.

(The above list was compiled in part from *Know Your Fats: The Complete Primer for Understanding the Nutrition of Fats, Oils, and Cholesterol* by Mary G. Enig, Ph. D.)

Trans Fat May Double
INFERTILITY RISKS!

A study found, "Each 2% increase in the intake of energy from trans unsaturated fats, as opposed to that from carbohydrates, was associated with a 73% greater risk of ovulatory infertility... Jorge E Chavarro, Janet W Rich-Edwards, Bernard A Rosner and Walter C Willett <u>Dietary fatty acid intakes and the risk of ovulatory infertility</u> *American Journal of Clinical Nutrition*, Vol. 85, No. 1, 231-237, January 2007

Cookies and Crackers Some packaged brands are loaded with trans fats—and just a few grams of these fats per day may double fertility risks. Chavarro's iron study found it's possible that trans fats contribute to inflammation and insulin problems, both drivers of infertility, he says. *Health.com Magazine* June, 2007. Page 80

13

Sugar

I know this is a book about trans fats and their debilitating affect on the human body. But I would be remiss if I didn't mention sugar since it too shares some similar negative affects in the body. The problem is sugar is hard to avoid unless you prepare meals from scratch with the appropriate ingredients.

Did you know that 95 percent of canned and processed products contain sugar? Did you know that 95 percent of canned and processed products contain sugar? That's right! Did you also know that the average American consumes 149 pounds of refined sugar each year? That is equivalent to 79 pounds of fat. No wonder so many people are overweight and having trouble losing the excess weight!! There was once a time when sweets were reserved for a once in a while indulgence, but now, they are a daily expectation. My goal in this chapter is to share from my teaching and master's training experiences and to highlight for you several reasons why sugar, like trans fat, is bad for your body.

Sugar depletes the body of B-complex vitamins, zinc, and the essential minerals, calcium and magnesium. First and foremost, sugar depletes the body of B-complex vitamins, zinc, and the essential minerals, calcium and magnesium. These vitamins and minerals are required for the digestion of sugar, both natural and refined. Complex carbohydrates like fruits, vegetables, and starches contain enough of the nutrients to assist our bodies in their own digestion. However, refined sugar has virtually none of these nutrients and requires them from the body's tissue stores to complete the digestive process. B-complex vitamins are taken from the nervous system while calcium and magnesium are robbed from the bones and teeth. In his book *Healthy Habits*, Dr. Tessler comments, "Consequently, refined sugar 'rips you off' of these needed nutrients resulting in 'raw' nerves." So when we are reaching for that cookie, piece of candy, or pancakes loaded with syrup, we are stealing from our bodies. When bones and teeth are leeched for their calcium and magnesium, they become porous which allows minerals to leak out into the body. Eventually they settle in the joints causing the condition known as arthritis. Let me further explain how this happens in the body.

When we are reaching for that cookie, piece of candy, or pancakes loaded with syrup, we are stealing from our bodies.

If you look at the fat metabolic chart #1, page 28, you will notice that in order for metabolism to complete itself correctly, B-complex, zinc, and magnesium are required and that trans fat products inhibit the process leading to the production of arachidonic acid and subsequently, PG #2 which causes pain. Now look at Chart #2 page 29. Insulin is yet another ingredient that can inhibit the process and lead to this pain causing prostaglandin. If our diets are high in simple sugars, then the vitamins and minerals are inhibited allowing for dihomo-gamma-linolenic acid (DGLA) to take over the metabolism process creating arachidonic acid and PG#2 is the end result. This acid is what settles in joints leading to arthritic conditions.

Effect of Sugar on White Blood Cell Activity

Amount of Refined Sugar Consumed	The Number of Bacteria a WBC Can Process in ½ Hour	Decrease in Immunity
No Sugar	14	0%
6 tsp. = 8 oz of soft drink	10	25%
12 tsp. = frosted brownie	5.5	60%
18 tsp. = apple pie ala mode	2	85%
24 tsp. = banana split	1	92%
Uncontrolled Diabetic	1	92%

(Special Note: A 12-ounce can of soda contains 9 teaspoons of sugar. An 8-ounce serving of fruit-flavored yogurt contains almost as much.)

The second impact of sugar on our metabolism is its effect on our immune system. Take a look at the above chart. Notice the amount of bacteria that white blood cells can process in one half hour when no sugar is consumed. Now read down the column. It is amazing to me how much sugar truly shuts down our immune systems. No wonder you get sick — your body is fighting to digest sugar and not fight bacteria!

Sugar is responsible for causing symptoms of fatigue.

Finally, sugar is responsible for causing symptoms of fatigue. One of my friends is always tired and wonders why. Well, I know her diet. She consumes a lot of sugar and refined, packaged foods which we already know contain sugar. When she eats, she feels great. Her body is energized as the refined sugars go directly to her blood stream. What happens next is the body responds to this high by releasing large amounts of insulin to counteract all the sugar and stabilize the blood stream. The result is a crash in her energy levels leaving her fatigued. And unless she removes sugar from her diet, she will remain chronically tired.

Does this cycle happen when any type of sugar is consumed? The answer is, No, it does not. When we eat refined, simple carbohydrates, our bodies respond in this way. Not so with natural, complex carbohydrates. These are made of long chains of simple sugars which your body digests slowly releasing a more balanced sugar supply. Whatever your body doesn't immediately use is stored in the liver as glycogen to be used at a later time. These are the sugars we need to be consuming saving the refined type for a truly special occasion.

At one point in my life I was facing so many health challenges like insomnia, severe hip and leg pain, swelling in my calf, neck pain, and when I walked my left leg was in such pain. At Dr. Bob's suggestion, I made some major diet changes like getting pop and candy bars out of my life. I was a total sugar addict! the first week without sugar was hard, but little by little I started feeling better and seeing health results which encourage me to keep going. What a difference! I would strongly recommend everyone to change or modify their diet.

~Kim M. Jackson

At this point you are probably wondering how in the world you are going to start eliminating refined sugar from your diet. As a time-crunched mom who was concerned about what was going into my child's body, I determined to really work on this aspect of our lives and I will say that it took commitment. My time was stretched thin with a full-time job, graduate school and single parenting a busy child. So I started simply. I read labels checking to see if sugar was the first ingredient listed. If it was, I immediately put the item back on the shelf. Then I eliminated all the obvious sugar items like candy and cookies.

As far as the soda issue goes, it was never an issue with me, I was already a water drinker, but I did consume diet sodas containing aspartame and sucralose which I eventually eliminated. However for those of you who are still hooked on that liquid candy, let me give you a few pieces of information. In the 1950s, a serving size of soda was a six and one half ounce bottle. Today it is up to a twenty ounce bottle. A 7-11 store Double Gulp is 64 ounces. That's potentially 600 empty calories!! You receive absolutely no nutritional value from that. Imagine how much better your body would feel if the Double Gulp consumers changed from soda to water. And think of the

We need to lose the soda habit and create a water habit.

money saved! I remember as a kid having to share a 16 ounce bottle of soda with my sister and brother. Now when we get together, there are liters of different sodas. We need to lose the soda habit and create a water habit.

The next phase for me was experimenting in recipes with alternatives to sugar like brown rice syrup and barley malt syrup. I used to use a sugar substitute in my mocha, but eventually after I learned more, I switched to using stevia, a sweet South American herb. Now, when you embark on this transformation in your lives, be aware of the different types of sugar alternatives and substitutes. What you DON'T want is another type of refined sugar and unfortunately they are readily

What you want is a naturally occurring sweetener like honey and maple syrup.

available and can fool the average consumer. If it is refined and synthetic, it will be no different than adding a chemical to your body and you know by now that these too will inhibit correct fat metabolism. Those ending in "-ol" are sugar alcohols. Also, be aware of evaporated cane juice and cane juice crystals

which are still sugar and can therefore cause challenges. What you want is a naturally occurring sweetener. In actuality these natural products, like honey and maple syrup, were the original sweeteners before sugar refining created a mass market product.

The bottom line is to try different alternatives. Experiment a little bit. Go to a whole food grocery store and ask them for recommendations. They have products on the shelf that use alternatives. Find what works for you and what you like. Will you have to experiment a bit? Probably. I once made a batch of chocolate chip cookies with grain sweetened chips and barley malt for the sugar. I don't think the dog would have eaten them. So don't be frustrated with the failures. Just keep on trying. Think about going through this transition with a friend. Not only is it more fun, but you can then split the cost of all those experimental recipes!

The information received from Dr. DeMaria encourages you make a choice as to what you want to put into your body. When I first came to the office I had back pain, digestive problems and some sinus problems. I took Pepto Bismol and Rolaids regularly. I now make conscious decisions reducing my sugar intake and am aware of my general eating habits. I have greatly reduced my fast food consumption. The most challenging change for me has been to decrease my "pop" intake, but after cutting back, the desire is diminishing.

~Drew Birdsall

Your body can't produce enough digestive enzymes without the right balance of minerals and B vitamins. Compensating for your sweet tooth by consuming extra healthy foods may be a losing battle since your body is no longer digesting or assimilating food efficiently. **This is another real challenge for children with hyperactivity, since they are already consuming food that is nutritionally stripped.**

> **Notice**
> ☑ **Eating sugar puts stress on digestion**
> ☑ **Poor digestion can lead to allergies**
> ☑ **Sugar consumption results in poor health**

Sweeteners To Avoid

☑ What about other refined sugars? **Brown sugar** is simply refined sugar that is sprayed with molasses to make it appear more whole. **Turbinado sugar** gives the illusion of health, but is just one step away from white sugar. Tubinado is made from 95 percent sucrose (table sugar). It skips only the final filtration stage of sugar refining, resulting in little difference in nutritional value.

☑ **Corn syrup** is found everywhere. It is used in everything from bouillon cubes to spaghetti sauce and even in some "natural" juices. Corn syrup processed from cornstarch is almost as sweet as refined sugar and is absorbed quickly by your blood. Corn-derived sweeteners pose other problems: they often contain high levels of pesticide residues that are genetically modified and are common allergy producers. This is a cheap and plentiful sweetener often used in soft drinks, candy and baked goods. Corn syrup is very similar to refined sugar in composition as well as effect.

☑ **Aspartame**, which is a common synthetic sweetener, affects the nervous system and brain in a very negative way. Aspartame is made from two proteins, or amino acids, which gives it its super sweetness. Aspartame has many harmful effects: behavior changes in children, headaches, dizziness, epileptic-like seizures and bulging of the eyes to name a few. Aspartame is an "excitotoxin", a substance that over stimulates neurons and causes them to die suddenly (as though they were excited to death). One of the last steps of aspartame metabolism is formaldehyde. The next time you consume diet soda, think. You are literally embalming yourself.

☑ **Sucrose** is found in white sugar and maple syrup. Sucrose requires very little digestion and provides instant energy followed by plummeting blood sugar levels. It stresses the entire body system.

☑ **Glucose** is also called dextrose. When combined with sucrose, glucose subjects your blood sugar to the same up and downs. In whole food form, it's in starches like beans and whole grain breads; they are also rich in soluble fiber—glucose takes longer to digest, resulting in more balanced energy.

☑ **Sorbitol, Mannitol & Xylitol** are synthetic sugar alcohols. Although these can cause less of an insulin jump in glucose to sugar, many people suffer gastric distress. You see these sugars listed as ingredients in foods.

☑ **Unrefined cane juice.** This is sugarcane in crystal form. Nothing more, nothing less. Unrefined cane juice is brown and granulated, contains 85 percent to 96.5 percent sucrose, and retains all of sugarcane's vitamins, minerals and other nutrients. Cane juice has a slightly stronger flavor and less intense sweetness than white sugar. Look for the brand names Sucanat® and Florida Crystals®.

☑ **Crystalline fructose.** This refined simple sugar has the same molecular structure as fruit sugar. It's almost twice as sweet as white sugar, yet releases glucose into the bloodstream much more slowly. Extra sugar gets stored in your liver as glycogen instead of continuing to flood your bloodstream. Thus, crystalline fructose appeals to diabetics and hypoglycemics.

The Best of the Naturals

Become sugar savvy! The term "natural," as applied to sweeteners, can mean many things. The sweeteners recommended below will provide you with steady energy because they take a long time to digest. Natural choices offer rich flavors, vitamins and minerals, without the ups and downs of refined sugars.

Sugar substitutes were actually the natural sweeteners of days past, especially honey and maple syrup. In health food stores, be alert for sugars disguised as "evaporated cane juice" or "cane juice crystals." These can still cause problems, regardless what the health food store manager tells you. My patients have seen huge improvements by changing their sugar choices.

☑ **Brown rice syrup.** Your bloodstream absorbs this balanced syrup, high in maltose and complex carbohydrates, slowly and steadily. Brown rice syrup is a natural for baked goods and hot drinks: it adds subtle sweetness and a rich, butterscotch-like flavor. To get sweetness from starchy brown rice, the magic ingredients are enzymes, but the actual process varies depending on the syrup manufacturer. "Malted" syrups use whole, sprouted barley to create a balanced sweetener. Choose these syrups to make tastier muffins and cakes. Cheaper, sweeter rice syrups use isolated enzymes and are a bit harder on blood sugar levels. For a healthy treat, drizzle gently heated rice syrup over popcorn to make natural caramel corn. Store in a cool, dry place.

☑ **Devansoy**™ is the brand name for powdered brown rice sweetener, which contains the same complex carbohydrates as brown rice syrup and a natural plant flavoring.

> Use barley malt syrup to add molasses-like flavor and light sweetness to beans, cookies, muffins and cakes.

☑ **Barley malt syrup.** This sweetener is made much like rice syrup, but it uses sprouted barley to turn grain starches into a complex sweetener that is digested slowly. Use barley malt syrup to add molasses-like flavor and light sweetness to beans, cookies, muffins and cakes. Store in a cool, dry place.

☑ **Amasake** is an ancient, oriental whole grain sweetener made from cultured brown rice. It has a thick, pudding-like consistency. Baked goods benefit from amasake's subtle sweetness, moisture and leavening power.

☑ **Stevia** is a sweet South American herb that has been used safely by many cultures for centuries. Extensive

> Stevia is 150 to 400 times sweeter than white sugar, has no calories and can actually regulate blood sugar levels.

scientific studies back-up these ancient claims to safety. However, the FDA has approved it only when labeled as a dietary supplement, not as a sweetener. Advocates consider stevia to be one of the healthiest sweeteners as well as a tonic to heal the skin. Stevia is 150 to 400 times sweeter than white sugar, has no calories and can actually regulate blood sugar levels. Unrefined stevia has a molasses-like flavor; refined stevia (popular in Japan) has less flavor and nutrients.

☑ **Fruitsource®.** This brand-name sweetener combines the sweetness of grape juice concentrate with the complex carbohydrates of brown rice syrup. *FruitSource* is light amber in color and 80 percent as sweet as white sugar. *Liquid Plus*, a similar product, better matches the sweetness of white sugar. Look for *FruitSource* in liquid and granulated form. Whichever form you choose, the options are better for your blood sugar than refined sugar!

☑ **Whole fruit.** For baking, try fruit purees, dried fruit and cooked fruit sauces or butters. The less water remaining in a fruit, the more concentrated its flavor and sugar content. You'll find fiber and naturally-balanced nutrients in whole fruits like apples, bananas and apricots. To add mild sweetness and moisture to baked goods, mix in the magic of mashed winter squashes, sweet potatoes and carrots!

☑ **Fructose** in whole foods provides balanced energy.

☑ **Honey.** It takes one bee an entire lifetime to produce a single tablespoon of honey from flower nectar. But that small amount goes a long way! Honey is mostly made of glucose and fructose and is up to twice as sweet as white sugar. Honey enters the bloodstream rapidly. Look for raw honey, which still contains some vitamins, minerals, enzymes and pollen. Honeys vary in color (according to their flower source) and range in strength from mild clover to strong orange blossom. A benefit of eating honey produced in your geographical region is that it may reduce hay fever and allergy symptoms by bolstering your natural immunity. Note: raw honey can lead to a toxic, sometimes fatal form of botulism in

> **It takes one bee an entire lifetime to produce a single tablespoon of honey from flower nectar.**

children under one. Limit honey consumption, as it results in similar results as sucrose.

☑ **Maltose** is the primary sugar in brown rice and barley malt syrups. Maltose is a complex sugar that is digested slowly. It is the sugar with "staying power."

☑ **Maple Syrup.** It takes about 10 gallons of maple sap to produce 1 gallon of maple syrup. Like honey, a little goes a long way. Maple syrup is roughly 65 percent sucrose and contains small amounts of trace minerals. Maple syrup has a rich taste and is absorbed fairly quickly into the bloodstream. Select real maple syrup that has no added corn syrup. Also, look for syrups that come from organic producers who don't use formaldehyde to prolong sap flow. Grade A syrups come from the first tapping: they range in color from light to dark amber. Grade B syrups come from the last tapping; they have more minerals and a stronger flavor and color.

> Select real maple syrup that has no added corn syrup.

☑ **Date sugar.** This sweetener is made from dried, ground dates, is light brown and has a sugary texture. Date sugar retains many naturally-occurring vitamins and minerals, is 65 percent sucrose and has a fairly rapid effect on blood sugar. Use it in baking instead of brown sugar, but reduce your baking time or temperature in order to prevent premature browning. Store in a cool, dry place.

☑ **Concentrated fruit juice.** All concentrates are not created equally. Highly-refined juice sweeteners are labeled "modified." These sweeteners, similar to white sugar, have lost both their fruit flavor and their nutrients. Better choices are fruit concentrates that have been evaporated in a vacuum. These retain rich fruit flavors and aromas and many vitamins and minerals. Carefully read labels on cereal, cookie, jelly and beverage containers, then choose products with the highest percentage of real fruit juice. Beware of white grape juice concentrates that aren't organic; their pesticide residues can be high!

☑ **Blackstrap molasses.** Molasses, a by-product of sugar production, is a highly-processed simple sugar that enters the bloodstream rapidly. Molasses may also contain chemical residues associated with the growing and refining of white sugar. If you grew up on conventional molasses, your taste buds may have to adjust to the softer bite of **blackstrap molasses, which contains high amounts of balancing minerals such as calcium, iron, potassium, magnesium, zinc, copper and chromium.** Use it as a sweetener in cakes, pies and cookies. Barbados molasses is sweeter and more syrupy than blackstrap; it is perfect for baking but lacks blackstrap's minerals. (Note: Diabetics should not use any type of molasses.)

Sugar Substitution

Amount Indicates the Equivalent of 1 Cup of White Sugar

Sweetener	Amount	Liquid Reduction	Suggested Use
Honey	1/2 - 2/3 cup	1/4 cup	All-purpose
Maple syrup	1/2 - 3/4 cup	1/4 cup	Baking & desserts
Maple sugar	1/2 - 1/3 cup	None	Baking & candies
Barley malt syrup	1 - 1 1/2 cups	1/2 cup	Breads & baking
Rice syrup	1 - 1/3 cups	1/2 cup	Baking & cakes
Date sugar	2/3 cup	None	Breads & baking
Blackstrap Molasses	1/2 cup	1/4 cup	Breads & baking
Fruit juice concentrate	1 cup	1/3 cup	All-purpose
Stevia	1 tsp/cup of water	1 cup	Baking

(Note: If you have a serious blood sugar regulation problem, such as diabetes or hypoglycemia, see your Health Care Practitioner to determine the type and amount of sweeteners your body can handle.)

14

Fats: Which to Cook or Not to Cook? That is the Question.

W hen it comes to cooking, oils and fats are not all created equal. You know by now that if the fat is hydrogenated or partially hydrogenated you should never consider them and you should remember that the Omega-3 fats should never be heated because their molecular structure is not stable enough. So what about everything else and those in between? My goal is to give you a guide to which oils you can safely use including which are heat tolerant.

Replacing trans fat has become quite the trick for the American food industry. Trans fat holds up well and can be heated over and over again saving restaurants a bundle on their fried offerings. And did I mention it is really cheap? However, its negative effects on your health are far from cheap. So what can you use when you bake or fry? In the world of frying, I just can't give the stamp of approval on deep fried products. They are simply too laden with fat and empty calories for me to justify in my diet. But if you **must** fry or sauté, you need to choose oil that is low in polyunsaturated fats and very heat tolerant meaning it has a high smoke factor and can be heated to high temperatures without breaking down and mutating into something very different! One of your best bets, and the original fats of choice of our grandparents, is animal fats which are very chemically stable due to their amounts of saturated fat. And yes, animal fats contain cholesterol, infamous as a cause for heart attacks. However, the correlation between dietary cholesterol and blood serum cholesterol is very weak according to tfX, a UK health watchdog. The danger with animal fats is that they are a fat that readily stores in our cells when taken in excess. Another good bet for baking and frying are your tropical oils which are also saturated and as a result, very stable when subjected to heat. These oils received a bad rap in the 1980s despite the protests of the US Surgeon General C. Everett Koop. He "dismissed the anti-tropical oil arguments as ill-founded and absurd" according the article "Alternatives to Trans Fats" printed by tfX. It was after that point that hydrogenated and partially hydrogenated vegetable oils, primarily from soy, entered the mainstream market and moved to center stage. The World Health Organization, WHO, claims that tropical oils have been given an unfair stigmatism despite their health benefits such as being a good source of lauric acid (the protective substance in mother's milk), being lower in energy content than any oil making it less fattening, protecting against heart disease and cancer, and having loads of antioxidants, to list a few. But WHO does not suggest a mass switch to tropical oils since it may disrupt the biodiversity of tropical forests already being ravaged. Incidentally, I used coconut oil once as a Crisco substitute in frosting for a cake. While I noticed the texture being slightly less creamy, no one else seemed to notice. So, on those rare and special occasions when you must bake or fry, you have a couple options other than the can of white stuff. But bake or fry sparingly — no one needs the extra calories or fat!

Olive oil, a monounsaturated oil, is another great option for both cooking and eating. It is very low in saturated fat, making it a much healthier alternative but not very suitable for high heat. Olive oil can tolerate temperatures of up to 350 degrees before breaking down, so it is perfect for light sautéing and baking. I use a Misto oil sprayer full of olive oil to coat pans before cooking just about everything and it really works well in keeping foods from sticking while adding a nice touch of flavor. But honestly, I live for olive oil on salads. Maybe it's because of my Italian heritage, but I will take a salad dressed in olive oil, balsamic or red wine vinegar, and sea salt and pepper any day over bottled dressing. My great grand-mother used to always make salads that way, with lots of olive oil, a little vinegar and a lot of salt. Give it a try!

There are a few things to know about olive oils before you buy them randomly. You want to purchase extra-virgin olive oil. It is the oil from the first pressing of the olives and it is rich in antioxidants and polyphenols which "are a tonic to cardiovascular health" (Hendley). This oil is the fruitiest and finest of the olive oils with a low level of acidity. Its color should be slightly green. You also want a cold pressed extra-virgin olive oil. This simply means that no chemical has been added to the extraction process, just good old pressure. Any Mediterranean country produces a good olive oil and even California produces good olive oil. None are better than another; it is all a matter of preference of taste.

Let's talk about flax oil next. Because this omega-3 fat is not heat tolerant and must be kept refrigerated due to its high polyunsaturated fat content, this nutty tasting oil is great for using on salads or even for dipping vegetables or breads for a once in a while treat. As a mom and daughter concerned for her family's health, I have had to be creative in getting flax oil into my family's diet. Since it can be a tough concept to, quite literally, swallow, I began using it in homemade salad dressings replacing part of other oils. It adds a rich smoothness to dressings and your whole family can reap the benefits of the omega-3 nutrients!! And quite honestly, when I tossed a salad for my parents using flax oil, they didn't even notice until I said something.

If you go to the grocery store and grab a bag of chips with no trans fat in them, you will probably notice that the oil used to cook the potatoes is either safflower or sunflower oil. These two oils do provide the opportunity to still eat your snack foods without also eating trans fat. Before I go further, let me clarify that **I AM NOT** saying it is okay to consume snack foods continually just because there is no trans fat in them. Snack foods are usually high in empty calories and fats and are meant for once in while consumption. Safflower and sunflower oils are part of the omega-6 fats which do provide your body with heart-friendly oleic acid. Most of them have been genetically modified to contain high levels of oleic acid so the ingredients list may say high-oleic sunflower or safflower oil. It simply means that the seeds were given an overhaul of heart healthy oleic acid. **What is important to remember is that your body needs to have a balance between omega-6 and omega-3 fats, a 4:1 ratio.** In Chapter 10, "Winning the Pain Game", the challenges your body faces when this ratio is out of balance are discussed. So do be careful when choosing what fats to eat. The goal is balance for optimal health.

There are other commonly used oils on the market today such as soy, canola, and peanut oils and you will find them listed in abundance on the ingredients lists of snack food packages. Being low in polyunsaturated fats, these oils do have a high tolerance for heat which is why they are so popular in fried foods and they are relatively affordable, another reason for their popular use. Once again, these oils are part of the omega-6 family so over consumption, which we tend to do in America, puts the 4:1 ratio out of balance introducing challenges for the body to overcome.

Every week there are a plethora of new oils being created as "healthy" substitutes with focus on the word created. Our bodies were meant to eat from nature for optimal health. Countries that still follow this are the healthiest countries in the world! We in this nation focus too much on synthetics as substitutes for the real thing and partially hydrogenated fats are a perfect example. What was created as a safe and healthy substitute for natural fats like butter and tropical fats has turned into a deadly issue; there are no safe fake fats. A final word to the wise, beware of the words esterification or esterified. It means the fat has been altered and is no longer in its natural state resulting in your body's inability to recognize it and properly digest it. Start reading labels and ingredients lists on packages of foods you purchase from the grocery store. Or, better yet, start doing your own baking and making of snack foods. This way you control all the ingredients that go into the recipe!

What was created as a safe and healthy substitute for natural fats like butter and tropical fats has turned into a deadly issue; there are no safe fake fats.

15

Trans Fat-Free Foods

Breakfast Suggestions

You should avoid starting the day with sweets, syrups, or packaged foods.

Breakfast can come from any source other than from a package, a can, an envelope, a powder, etc. Breakfast will affect insulin levels in you which makes a major impact on the craving for sugar. You should avoid starting the day with sweets, syrups, or packaged foods. Rotating foods is important as well.

Avoid bananas, dates, figs, grapes and raisins in the morning.

So where do you start? Avoid bananas, dates, figs, grapes and raisins in the morning. These foods will raise insulin and cause blood sugar variations and can affect the production of prostaglandins. Use wholesome non-sugar breakfast cereals with rice, almond or oat milk.

You could bake a coconut. (Drill holes to let milk out; cook at 325 degrees for 10 minutes — mmmmmm good!) Don't limit yourself to traditional breakfast choices. Here are some suggestions for you to try:

➢ **Oatmeal** is a simple food. It takes less than seven minutes to prepare. Boil water; add the oats and sprinkle with Celtic Sea Salt® and possibly some homemade applesauce. You can add almonds or sesame seeds, great sources of calcium. Walnuts and pecans are excellent sources of omega-3 fats. Any other seeds that you like can be added.

➢ **Rice cakes** with almond butter, sesame butter or cashew butter are great options. Try no-sugar-added jellies and jams. Rice cakes do have a higher glycemic index so take note if blood sugar levels are an issue with you.

➢ **Multi-grain pancakes** made with water, rice, almond or oat milk are another option. Spread with jelly containing no sugar. Kids love it with applesauce and cinnamon. You could even try REAL maple syrup.

➢ **Breakfast cereals** with no partially hydrogenated oils or sugar make a great option, too.

➢ **Eggs** are an excellent source of protein and sulfur that is important for the production of collagen in the body.

➢ **Whole wheat bread** is definitely better than white bread. If wheat gluten causes digestive challenges for you, try a sprouted grain bread like Ezekiel Bread or spelt bread. You can find these options and others in the freezer section at your local whole foods market. Or make your own bread!

➢ **Minimal to no dairy** is best since dairy can alter the digestion of omega-3 fats. We tend to over eat dairy products which can cause chronic ear infections leading to prescriptions of antibiotics, something we need to avoid.

➢ **Pork** is not the other white meat. Whatever the pig eats, you eat. They wallow in mud among other materials and eat anything, healthy and toxic alike!

➢ **Yogurt** made from goat milk is a good protein source. Unfortunately it is hard to find yogurt without added sugars or cane juice. You can sweeten plain yogurt with a few raisins, cinnamon or even crushed almonds.

➢ **Cheese.** I would encourage you to use rice cheese. It is possible to buy pre-wrapped slices of rice cheese in a variety of flavors. Goat cheese, chevre, and feta are great options.

refrigerator in olive oil and even infuse it with flavors like herbs and sun-dried tomatoes.

> **Squash** can be eaten for breakfast! Bake it with cinnamon and your whole family will like it.

> **Juice.** I encourage my patients not to consume orange juice or grapefruit juice when the temperature is below 60 degrees as it can cause mucus formation leading to congestion. Your best bets are apple juice or pure cranberry juice, diluted.

> **Water** should be purified or from a quality spring. Check labels as some springs are not any better than tap water.

> **Meats** should be organic. You don't want the added antibiotics or growth hormones given to animals.

Lunch Suggestions

Packing lunches is an important part of a healthy lifestyle. This way you control what you and your family are eating. You can purchase antibiotic-free and nitrate-free lunch meats from whole foods markets and from many grocery store chains. Keep an eye on the condiments and avoid those with sugar or evaporated cane juice. You can substitute almond butter for the stand-by PB&J. Peanuts contain molds and yeast which can cause immune issues which is why I recommend almond butter. Vary your breads as well and stick to whole grains. And of course no snack foods cooked in or containing hydrogenated fats! Look for those made with safflower, olive, or sunflower oil.

We get antibiotic and nitrate-free turkey from the health food store. You can make almond butter and jelly sandwiches. Vary the bread and jelly. You can use pita bread, flat bread and any grain, but vary it. Make veggie salads, tuna salad, egg salad, turkey salad, chicken salad sandwiches with rice cheese, lettuce and safflower mayo or whatever condiment you prefer. Use rice cheese pizza, pizza bagels, almond butter on celery and other fresh cut up veggies. Make whole pasta with butter or nutmilk in a container that keeps the contents warm. **You must read all labels.**

No french fries cooked with partially hydrogenated fats.

Condiments containing no sugar or corn syrup are best purchased from a health food store. Most condiments today, including the major commercial brands, always seem to contain sugar hidden as organic evaporated cane juice crystals.

Dinner Suggestions

It is estimated that more than one-half of meals are eaten out of the home, including dinner.

Not having your family on medication for allergies alone should justify the additional time spent on food preparation. Dinner is a very interesting meal. Families rarely unite at the kitchen table for dinner as they have in the past. It is estimated that more than one-half of meals are eaten out of the home, including dinner.

You should have a family meeting to make decisions as to what type of food you would like to be preparing for your evening meals. Make it a fun, cooperative event where everyone participates, creating a unit for discussion and laughter.

You can eat anything you want *except* pork, hydrogenated fat, pre-packaged/powdered/boxed or canned food that contains preservatives and/or artificial colorings, flavorings, etc. We do eat meat (normally organic, antibiotic-free), but you do not have to have red meat with every meal. We utilize pastas, beans, legumes and a variety of casseroles.

I encourage you to purchase as much food as you can fresh, therefore after you are finished with a meal, instead of having it as a leftover, you could freeze it and have it at another time. I encourage individuals to pre-bake several meals prior to the beginning of the week. There are an enormous variety of foods that can be used, i.e., squashes, zucchini, eggplant, potatoes, yams as well as a variety of casseroles. In other words—make your food from scratch!

Your ethnic background and food taste will determine the type of foods you like to eat. Your goal is fresh, organic and alive food. Varying foods is important. In our household we use different organic tomato-based sauces, organic starter-type foods (organic broths).

BE CREATIVE! Canned and pre-packaged food are often mineral depleting, metabolism altering, toxin creating chemical time bombs.

You don't need to use or consume dessert. I'm not exactly sure where this habit started, however, ending a meal with sugar puts enormous stress on the liver, pancreas, and digestive system. Your body is busy breaking down simple carbohydrates and adding proteins to it can confuse the body. Utilizing and putting sugar on top of this causes an enormous overload on the pancreas.

You could find some of Grandma's old recipes and use them, but be cautious of the amount of sugar.

Salmon, tuna, eggs and chicken can all be used. There is even turkey bacon, and turkey, lamb and chicken sausage. Remember to read labels because some of those products contain unhealthy oils, sugar and preservatives.

I would encourage you to visit a bookstore, health food store and even the Internet for favorite recipes that you can utilize. There are many wonderful health magazines that have numerous recipes.

Sweet Suggestions

There are sources of naturally made cookies and desserts that can be purchased at your local health food store. We only have dessert on special occasions. We find recipes in various wholesome dessert books.

Amaranth is an ancient flour product that can be used in replacement of wheat. There are nut and grain ice creams. We have rave results every time we take apple crisp with home-churned ice cream to somebody's house.

Snacks

I encourage patients to consume a minimum of one apple, one carrot and a quart of water per day along with their other normal food choices. Having wholesome homemade snacks is ideal. By utilizing a food co-op, you can often purchase very good snacks that are made with the proper ingredients.

Keep cut-up vegetables and fruits on hand for yourself and family. *Consume fruits only on an empty stomach*, not after a meal.

Vary your snacks. There are healthy snack foods available without partially hydrogenated fats including cookies without sugar. Popcorn made with olive oil or an air popper is excellent.

Visit health food stores, look into a food co-op. You can find excellent baking mixes having very simple ingredients. Have your children bake with you. This is a great wintertime activity.

COST OF FOOD

Eating healthier will drastically reduce money spent stocking our medicine cabinets.

Consider your cost of over-the-counter medications—antacids, sinus medications and pain killers—to treat symptoms of improper eating. Eating healthier will drastically reduce money spent stocking your medicine cabinets.

I often hear individuals complain that it is expensive to eat healthy. Many health food stores today have competitive prices. The cost for organic food may be slightly higher than commercially prepared food due to supply and demand. Prices in health food stores, from my experience, usually are lower in the second part of the month. Attempt to buy food on sale. "European" grocery stores carry wonderful and healthy foods at a price far lower than health food stores. Utilize a food co-op. You can save hundreds of dollars every month. Find local food producers. During harvest time, you can freeze many of the foods. Living healthy requires some work and participation.

Compare how much money you spend every time you eat out versus making that same food at home. Although it takes time, remember we need to spend more time with each other than we have in the past.

16

The Transition

Have you ever heard the saying, "Good, better, best Never let it rest until good becomes better and better becomes best." This is the best approach to changing the way you and your family eat. Change will come, but it will come little by little. It is a process. The following are excellent transitional charts to assist you in making the transition from good to best. This information was taken in part from *Junk Food to Real Food, A Blueprint for Healthier Eating* by Carol A. Nostrand.

Transition Chart I

Food to Avoid PROTEINS	Food to Enjoy PROTEINS	
Eliminate Immediately	*Acceptable Foods* Experiment with These	*Vital Foods* Primarily Use These
Meats with additives, such as luncheon meat packed with nitrites (bologna, salami, etc.)	Meat without additives, hormones, antibiotics, etc., raised free-range on organic feed	Sprouts
Meat with hormones, etc.	Deep ocean or pure-lake fish	Fresh, raw nuts and seeds: flax, chia, pumpkin, sunflower, sesame, almond, pecan, brazil, walnut, filbert, etc.
Processed cheese		
Processed eggs	Nuts and grain as the source to make rice, almond milk, cheese, and yogurt	Nut butters
Processed chicken— raised in small coops, injected with antibiotics, etc.		Nut milks
	Goat's milk, chevre, feta cheese (Goat's milk is very close to human milk constituents) and is acceptable, but not daily.	Organic eggs
Pork		Beans: lentils, split peas, black beans, etc.
Pasteurized, homogenized cow's milk		
Yogurt with sugar, and toxic additives		

Transition Chart II

Food to Avoid CARBOHYDRATES	Food to Enjoy CARBOHYDRATES	
Eliminate Immediately	*Acceptable Foods* *Experiment with These*	*Vital Foods* *Primarily Use These*
Sugar: white, brown, turbinado, sucrose, glucose, corn syrup, fructose, etc.	Raw honey; blackstrap molasses; barley malt; pure maple syrup	Vegetables: squash, carrots, celery, tomatoes, beets, cabbage, broccoli, cauliflower, leeks, turnips, radish, lettuce, etc.
Chocolate	Carob	
Processed carbohydrates such as white flour and white flour products	Whole grain bread	Fruit: apples, pears, plums, etc.
White rice	Whole grain pasta	Sea vegetables
Anything packaged or canned with sugar, salt or toxic additives	Grain/Nut ice cream made without toxic additives or sugar	Whole grains: brown rice, millet, rye, barley, etc.
Processed pasta		
Ice cream with sugar and toxic additives		

Transition Chart III

Food to Avoid LIPIDS	Food to Enjoy LIPIDS	
Eliminate Immediately	*Acceptable Foods* *Experiment with These*	*Vital Foods* *Primarily Use These*
Oils that are rancid or overheated	High Oleic safflower, sunflower, olive oil	Raw, cold-processed oils: olive, sunflower, sesame, flax, almond, walnut, avocado
Rancid animal fats, such as lard, bacon drippings, etc.	Butter	Raw, unsalted butter
Anything deep-fat fried		Avocado
Artificially hardened fats, such as margarine and shortenings		Fresh, raw nuts and seeds

Transition Chart IV

Food to Avoid OTHER	Food to Enjoy OTHER	
Eliminate Immediately	*Acceptable Foods* *Experiment with These*	*Vital Foods* *Primarily Use These*
Coffee, tannic-acid teas; excess alcohol	Pure grain coffee substitutes	Herb teas and seasonings
Common table salt (sodium chloride)	Not more than one glass a day of non-chemicalized wine or beer	Organic apple cider vinegar
Any commercial condiments with sugar, salt or toxic additives	Aluminum-free baking powder	Home-made condiments without salt or sugar
Commercial soft drinks made with toxic additives and sugar	Soft drinks made without chemicals, sugar or toxic additives	Freshly juiced vegetables and fruits Fresh fruit ice cream
	Potassium balanced salt; celtic sea salt	Reverse osmosis purified water
	Vegetable salt and kelp	

17

The Best Food Pyramid

Recognizing that if America doesn't change their eating habits, "our children may be the first generation that cannot look forward to a longer life span than their parents", the government unveiled a new food pyramid discarding its former "one-size-fits-all" pyramid in the hopes that with new guidelines, America will become slimmer (USDA). The new guide spells out serving sizes and includes a recommended 30 minutes a day of exercise to reduce risks of chronic diseases and even be a preventative to these diseases. It is much more specific and can be tailored more individually simply by heading to its website, www.mypyramid.gov.

While this new food design is a good idea and the government should be applauded for their efforts, this new pyramid tap dances around the fact that we as a nation eat too much sugar. In an attempt to make their products more healthy and in closer compliance to this new pyramid, General Mills has overhauled their cereals to contain whole grains boldly stating, "The new food pyramid recommends more whole grain...and General Mills guarantees it in every box." And good for General Mills. But the fact still remains that their cereals still contain too much sugar!

While the pyramid is fine for the average American, it still has its shortcomings for athletes. Leslie Bonci, MPH, RD, LDN, director of Sports Nutrition at the University of Pittsburgh, says that for many of the professional athletes she counsels, the site is not specific enough. "My athletes don't want to dance around the subject," she says. "Their attitude is 'tell me when to eat; tell me what to eat; and tell me how much'."

In a statement from CSPI spokesperson Margo G. Wootan said, "The Dietary Guidelines unveiled in January were the strongest ever, but the new pyramid doesn't clearly communicate that advice to the public. By making "one size doesn't fit all" the mantra, and by replacing one pyramid with 12, the government has made this advice more complicated than it needs to be. There are simple key principles about healthy eating that truly do work for all Americans, and those could have been represented on one symbol.

Such a symbol would have made it immediately clear that we should be eating more fruits and vegetables; low-fat and fat-free dairy products as opposed to cheese and two percent milk; chicken and lean meats as opposed to hamburgers; whole grains as opposed to refined grains; and for everyone, less soda and less salt. But because one needs to go to a web site to get any of that detail, this new symbol is a missed opportunity. USDA seems to have bent over backward to avoid upsetting any particular commodity group or food company by not showing any foods that Americans should eat less of.

Fruit and Veggie Diet

Can a diet rich in fruits and vegetables keep you trim? Nutritionists say so, and now there's data to back them up.

Researchers tracked more than 74,000 women aged 38 to 63 for 12 years. Those who boosted their intake of fruits and vegetables by four servings a day had a 24 percent lower risk of obesity than those who cut their fruits and vegetables by about two servings a day.

What to do: Pack some baby carrots for snacks, start (or end) lunch with wedges of cantaloupe, serve at least two vegetables for dinner, etc. Who can complain about roasted asparagus, broccoli in garlic sauce, or sautéed spinach?

International Journal of Obesity
advance online publication, 5 October 2004.

The government should be using the dietary guidelines as a blueprint for national action and the basis for sound nutrition policies. How can parents effectively guide their kids' food choices when so much soda and junk food is for sale in America's schools, and with so many billions of dollars in junk food advertising aimed squarely at kids? How can people balance calories in with energy out without calorie counts on fast-food menu boards?

Whatever the content of the pyramid, the government does very little to help American's eat accordingly. If the government does with this pyramid what it did with the last one, which is to say very little, then we can expect a similar result: Americans will become fatter and will remain just as vulnerable to heart disease, cancer, and diabetes.

Now there's a mouthful!! My observation for the oil consumption portion of the pyramid, what this book is all about, is very vague. The pyramid creators feel we get enough oil in our diets. They sidestep the critical need for plant based omega-3 fats. The ADHD to Alzheimer's chapter is quite clear on that. Many if not most of our modern health issues are directly related to a lack of quality and quantity consumed levels of alpha linolenic acid precursor foods. I agree, we get enough oil, but it is mostly from man-made substitutes or omega-6 fats. Our current state of poor health in our society is directly linked to the "fat phobia", low-fat diet. I recommend omega-3 flax oil amounts based on the weight of a patient. Generally one tablespoon of organic, high lignan flax oil per one hundred pounds of body weight is my recommendation. The pyramid's recommendation of oil consumption is based on age. Trust me, a bigger individual requires more oil to function optimally in comparison to a smaller individual. One thing you need to remember, never heat omega-3 fats, including flax and canola oils. Use them cold.

The pyramid recognizes the need for a shift from refined grains to whole grains, which is a step in the right direction and I applaud them for this. But, be advised. The whole grains and the oils to prepare them as discussed in Chapter 10, "Winning the Pain Game", can lead to your painful tissue and obesity.

So what does the new pyramid look like? The picture below is an example of what an active 40 year old woman would need on a daily basis. Are you curious? Check it out at www.mypyramid.gov.

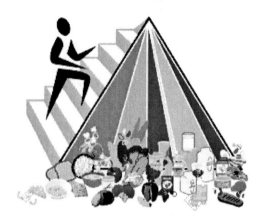

The Mediterranean Diet

At this point you may be slightly confused as to which pyramid is best. I can say that the healthiest diet in the world is the Mediterranean diet. The Mediterranean-style diet is the most successful for the greatest number of people. I would like all my patients to follow this plan and I do make this suggestion. It is steeped in fruits, vegetables, beans, nuts, olive oil, and more. Those on this diet experience fewer heart attacks and heart disease problems. Children on the Mediterranean diet will have reduced hyperactivity and will be less likely to develop heart disease. Scientists tracking the health benefits related to a diet concluded that all participants should be on the Mediterranean diet. After four years, those on this diet had two-thirds fewer heart attacks and one-third less hospitalizations for heart related problems. Remarkably, the cholesterol levels were about the same among those on the Mediterranean diet as those that were not following the plan, proving that cholesterol has little or nothing to do with heart attacks!

This is the pyramid that should be hanging in all doctor's offices!

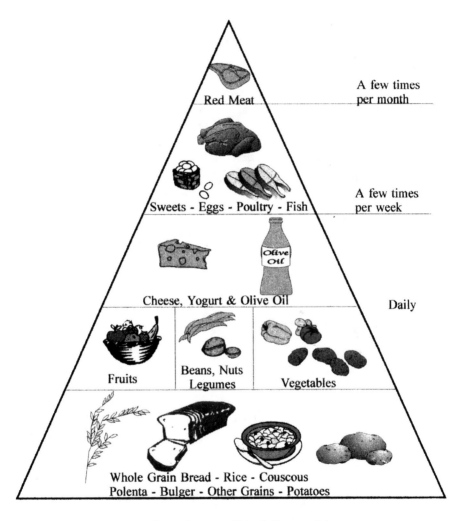

A few times per month

A few times per week

Daily

Red Meat

Sweets - Eggs - Poultry - Fish

Cheese, Yogurt & Olive Oil

Fruits

Beans, Nuts Legumes

Vegetables

Whole Grain Bread - Rice - Couscous
Polenta - Bulger - Other Grains - Potatoes

Mediterranean Food Pyramid

Mediterranean Mix

In a study of more than 22,000 adults in Greece, those who ate a more traditional Mediterranean diet had a lower death rate (largely due to fewer deaths from heart disease and cancer) than others. Participants got points for eating foods like vegetables, fruits, beans, fish and olive oil more often and for eating foods like meat and dairy products (which are rarely low-fat in Greece) less often. They also received points for consuming moderate amounts of alcohol. A lower death rate wasn't linked to any single food group.

What to do: It's possible that something else about the people who chose to eat a Mediterranean diet kept them alive longer. But there's plenty of evidence from other studies to recommend less fatty meat and dairy and more vegetables, fruits, beans, fish and unsaturated oils like olive and canola.

New England Journal of Medicine **348: 2599, 2595, 2003**

The Best Meds

In an Italian study of 180 people with the metabolic syndrome, those who ate a healthy Mediterranean diet had less inflammation and insulin resistance.

Patients on the Mediterranean diet ate twice as much fruit, vegetables, beans, nuts, whole grains, olive oil, and omega-3 fats (largely from fish) — and half as much saturated fat — as the control group. Both groups consumed roughly equal amounts of alcohol, total fat, protein, and carbohydrates.

After two years, signs of insulin resistance and inflammation (like C-reactive protein and interleukin-6) were lower and blood vessels were more flexible in the Mediterranean dieters than in the control group.

What's more, the Mediterranean group improved more than the control group on all measures of the metabolic syndrome — large waist size, low HDL ("good") cholesterol, and higher-than-optimal blood sugar, blood pressure, and triglycerides.

What to do: Eat more fruits, vegetables, beans, whole grains, and seafood. Replace saturated fats from meat and dairy with unsaturated fats from oils and nuts.

J. Amer. Med. Assoc. **292: 1440, 2004**

RESOURCES

Biotics Research Corporation has a solid clinical reputation for excellence. I use their oils and other products in my practice and for my personal and family use.

Biotics Research Corporation
www.bioticsresearch.com

Biotics Research is a family-owned and operated whole food supplement manufacturer the sells exclusively to healthcare professionals. They utilize their own on-site laboratories for researching and developing the highest quality, most efficacious nutritional supplements for proven results. Their products range from emulsified vitamins and minerals for optimal absorption, to glandular products for optimal endocrine support. Biotics also have a full line of essential fatty acid products including both liquid and solid forms of omegas.

About Biotics Research Corporation

At Biotics Research Corporation, we manufacture our own products on-site, in our own state-of-the-art facilities, allowing for complete control of the entire manufacturing process. In our on-site laboratories, the highly skilled members of our Quality Control Team, utilize modern, sophisticated technologies and validated analytical methods to test incoming raw materials, monitor manufacturing processes, perform in-process testing, and test all finished products prior to their release for shipment. In fact, many aspects of our cGMPs (current Good Manufacturing Practices) exceed the new, recently enacted FDA guidelines for dietary supplements in order to ensure the safety and effectiveness of our products.

Quality Control has the authority to approve and/or reject all specifications and procedures associated with the production and release of all raw materials, packaging materials and finished products, including test methods and results, instrument calibrations, and processing records. QC conducts all internal audits, and validates and audits all raw material and packaging suppliers and service vendors as well.

All incoming raw materials are subject to appropriate testing prior to their release for production. Tests conducted include: identity, potency, biological activity, microbiological including bacteria, yeast and mold (including aflatoxins), heavy metals (arsenic, cadmium, lead & mercury), pesticides, and residual chemical solvents. Retained samples are maintained of all raw materials and finished products for future testing requirements (raw material stability & finished product expiration date verification).

All bulk finished products (tablets & capsules) are inspected and are subjected to metal detection prior to their being sampled by QC. They are then subject to appropriate disintegration and/or dissolution testing, and potency testing prior to being released to packaging. All liquid and powder products are tested for potency prior to packaging as well. Finally, microbiological testing is performed on all packaged finished product, and document reconciliation is completed prior to their being released for shipping.

All testing is performed by our trained QC personnel using state-of-the-art laboratory instrumentation based on common methods including High Performance Liquid Chromatography, Inductively Coupled Plasma-Optical Emission Spectroscopy, Atomic Absorption Spectroscopy, Fourier Transform Infrared Spectroscopy, Ultra-Violet/Visible Spectroscopy, Thin Layer Chromatography and Gas Chromatography-Mass Spectrometry and Gel Electrophoresis.

Unlike many companies that are struggling to meet the new GMP requirements established by the FDA, companies that are being regulated into implementing quality programs, extensive Quality Control has always been part of the corporate fabric of Biotics Research Corporation.

From day one, the mantra of Biotics Research Corporation has been "Innovation and Quality". Our goals remain unchanged – utilize innovative ideas and carefully researched concepts with advanced techniques to develop products of superior quality and effectiveness – bringing you "The Best of Science and Nature".

Visit us online at www.bioticsresearch.com

Mediterranean Food Pyramid 134

Mental issues 92

Metabolic problems 92

Mineral deficiencies 77

Minerals 77

Misinterpretation of fat 17

Modifying diet 8

Molasses 108

Monosaturated fats 18-19, 50, 61

Monounsaturated oil 112

Myelin sheath 84

N

Natural fat 52

Natural practitioners 10

Natural sweeteners 104

Nutrition Facts panel 68

O

Oatmeal 58

Obesity 2, 65

Oleic acid 19

Oleo margarine 46

Olive oil 112

Omega-3 41, 50, 74

Omega-6 43, 74

Oppositional Defiant Disorder (ODD) 81

Optimal female health 9

Over-processed foods 36

Oxidation 50

P

Pain relievers 91

Partial hydrogenation 63

Peanuts 119

Percent Daily Value (%DV) 68

Pharmaceutical companies 3

Physically altered fats 67

Polyphenols 113

Polyunsaturated fat 20, 61

Pork 118

Post-surgical infections 5

Precursor foods 34

Prednisone 35

Progesterone deficiency 4

Prostaglandin 1 (PG1) 27, 73

Prostaglandin 2 (PG2) 27, 73

Prostaglandin 3 (PG3) 34, 73

Prostaglandins 27, 34, 62, 73, 75
    table 77

R

Red meat 3

Refined sugar 98

Resources 135

Ritalin 81

S

Safflower oil 74

Salmon capsules 35, 63

Salmon oil 43, 63

Saturated fat 13, 55

Saturated fat molecules 18

Schedule II drug 82

Scurvy 5

Seniors 85

Serving size 66, 129

Sjoren's syndrome 92

Skin problems 92

Snacks, healthy 122

Soda 83

Sorbitol 103

Spoilage 47

Statins 4, 57

Steroid 35

Sterol 55

Stevia 101, 105

Sucralose 100

Sucrose 103

Sugar 23, 83, 99
    effect on white blood cells 99
    promoting inflammation 57

Sugar alcohols 101

Sugar alternatives 101

Sugar substitution 101, 109

Summary of ADHD to Alzheimer's 86

Summary of alpha-linolenic acid 37

Summary of cholesterol 59

Summary of non-essential arachidonic acid 38

Summary of trans fats 64, 94

Sunflower oil 74

Supplement Facts panel 69

Sweet suggestions 121

Sweeteners to avoid 102

Sweeteners, natural 104

Synthetic vitamins 36

T

Tingling in extremities 92

Trans fat 2, 25, 46, 64, 66, 84, 89
    adverse effects of 95
    half life of 66
    per serving 66

Trans fat summary 64, 94

Trans fat-free foods 117

Transition Charts
    I 125
    II 126
    III 126
    IV 127

Tropical oil 112

Turbinado sugar 102

U

Urinary problems 92

V

Vioxx 27

Vitamin B 77

Vitamin deficiencies 77

Vitamins
  synthetic 36

W

Wall Street 10

White blood cell activity 99

Whole Foods Market 10

Whole fruit 106

X

Xylitol 103

Also available from Dr. Robert DeMaria ...

DVDs, Power Point Presentations

- A one-hour DVD with Dr. Bob on ADHD for $43.50.
- Dr. Bob's ADHD Power Point Slides for Presentation on CD for $33.50.
- Combined DVD & the Power Point Slides on CD together for just $56.50.

An order form for these & many other items is included on page 147.

<u>Distance Learning Workshops - CD</u>

Product Description	Price/Unit	Quantity	Total
Alzheimer's, ADHD & Depression	$ 9.95	_____	_____
Breast Cancer Pattern	9.95	_____	_____
Cholesterol – The True Facts	9.95	_____	_____
Clearing Skin Body Spots	9.95	_____	_____
Dispelling the Joy of Soy Myth	9.95	_____	_____
Hair Analysis	9.95	_____	_____
HRT – A Drugless Approach	9.95	_____	_____
Improving Memory	9.95	_____	_____
Improving Your Immune System	9.95	_____	_____
Joint Pain & Stiffness Help w/o Meds	9.95	_____	_____
Lose Weight with Fat Flush	9.95	_____	_____
Osteoporosis	9.95	_____	_____
Pain Relieving Meal Planning	9.95	_____	_____
Teeth Tell a Lot	9.95	_____	_____
Thyroid Advanced	9.95	_____	_____
Thyroid Basic – Hypothyroid	9.95	_____	_____
Trans Fat	9.95	_____	_____
Understanding the Yeast Connection	9.95	_____	_____
Whole Food B Vitamins	9.95	_____	_____
Winning the Pain Game	9.95	_____	_____
Why Am I So Tired?	9.95	_____	_____

Sub $_____

Ohio Residents add 6.75% Sales Tax $_____

TOTAL (SEE "ORDER FORM" ON PAGE 147) $_____

An order form for these workshops & many other items is included on page 147.

Special Appearances
Radio, TV &
Corporate Events

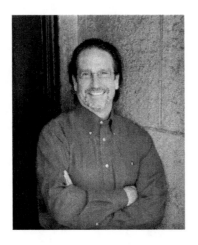 Dr. DeMaria is available on a limited basis to speak at your next Corporate Event or Convention. His energetic speaking style will inspire, educate and motivate your employees or downline to greater levels of health, wealth and personal confidence. Dr. Bob's enthusiasm for life is **contagious**!

To schedule or inquire please call:

1.888.922.5672

or email: drbob@druglessdoctor.com

Books by Dr. Bob

Dr. Bob's Drugless Guide to Detoxification

This may be the most toxic time in history. Daily headlines report the negative conditions of our water, food, and air. The "green movement" is popularly creating a mindset to secure a safe cleaner environment, but little is said about the circumstances our bodies need to contend with. This book is a logical plan that establishes true wellness in your body from the inside out. Dr. Bob shares clinically proven, time-tested protocols that can be followed in the comfort of your own home—no need to travel to expensive clinics or follow strict and stressful diet plans.

You will learn what to purchase at your own grocery store to maintain a healthy body; be empowered to make wise choices and not be dependent on medications; avert possible surgical intervention to remove an exhausted dysfunctional organ; and learn what to eat and what to avoid to create and optimally functioning cellular environment!

Dr. Bob's Drugless Guide to Balancing Female Hormones

The time tested information is this book is designed to create a state of optimal health in the female hormonal system. Dr. Bob's insight into cell function will empower the reader to make wise choices designed to nourish and detoxify the body with items that can be easily incorporated in a day to day routine. You will learn that a clear and clean lymphatic system is important and that a functioning liver is vital for balance. The role of nutrients like iodine and proper oil help create the foundation needed to progress into hormonal maturity without annoying body signals. You will be exposed to the procedures that Dr. Bob has used in his career transition his patients to feeling great without medication.

Dr. Bob's Guide to
Stop ADHD in 18 Days

A Drugless Family Guide to Optimal Health

SEE IF YOU CAN PASS THE ADHD TEST ON PAGE 8. Anyone can successfully overcome ADHD and Hyperactivity without drugs. This book details how to get your children and family off medications and detrimental junk foods filled with trans-fatty acids, dairy products, sugar and preservatives, so that they can have optimal, natural health. This is a simple, effective step by step plan that includes adding FLAX OIL, modifying your diet and vitamin/ mineral intake. The protocol will improve your nervous system function; help you overcome behavioral and learning problems. It will improve insomnia, mood swings and irritability. The result will be your body healing itself naturally. Participants in the pilot program saw improvement in only 18 days. NATURALLY!!!

Dr. Bob's Trans Fat
Survival Guide:

Why No Fat, Low Fat, Trans Fat is KILLING YOU!!

This book explains the dangers of trans fat, commonly called hydrogenated and partially hydrogenated fat, as well as how to recognize them in every day foods by properly reading nutritional labels. Along with trans fat, you will learn the different types of fats, which ones are beneficial, and which ones should be used for cooking, baking or eating. Not to leave the reader hanging with questions on how to eliminate dangerous fats and take on a healthier approach to life, there are several sections dealing with how to make those changes, transitioning healthier foods into their eating plan. This book will encourage and empower you to make better choices and learn to live an optimal and healthy life.

Dr. Bob's Guide to Optimal Health

A God-Inspired, Biblically-Based
12 Month Devotional to Natural Health Restoration

The Guide to Optimal Health is a Spirit of the Lord inspired collection of natural health tips. There are 365 daily tips designed to slowly transform your life to the finest health. Experience suggests that it may take up to twenty-one days to create a new habit. The first of 18 different patterns discussed is water. There are twenty-one daily natural health tips and associated Bible verses focusing on water. There is a daily **Natural Prescription for Health.** At the end of the Guide there are several reference tables including a Food Combining Chart, Glycemic Index, a Good and Not So Good Sweeteners, a pH Chart, and a Transition Food Guide. The material you will learn will empower you to make choices that will have eternal impact on you, your family and friends.

Dr. Bob & Debbie's Guide to Sex and Romance

Dr. Bob and Debbie's Guide to Sex and Romance is a collection of personal and clinical based evidence including protocols applied and successfully used from Dr. Bob's healthcare practice. Dr. Bob and Debbie also share from their common sense experience from forty years of their personal relationship and over thirty years of marriage. You will gain from the insight they have gleaned from their involvement and observations discovered while being in natural health since 1978. The DeMaria's have watched the decline of the overall personal health of the new patients presented to the clinic and discuss the restoration of those individuals overall health in the guide. Dr. Bob linked the associated deterioration of sexual desire and whole body dysfunction with patients having chronic health challenges.